DECISION MAKING IN
Dental Treatment Planning

DECISION MAKING IN

Dental Treatment Planning

Walter B. Hall, A.B., D.D.S., M.S.D.

Professor and Chairman
Department of Periodontics
University of the Pacific School of Dentistry
San Francisco, California

W. Eugene Roberts, D.D.S., Ph.D.

Professor and Chairman
Department of Orthodontics
Indiana University School of Dentistry
Indianapolis, Indiana

Eugene E. LaBarre, B.A., D.M.D., M.S.

Professor and Chairman
Department of Removable Prosthodontics
University of the Pacific School of Dentistry
San Francisco, California

Artwork by
Eric Curtis, D.D.S.
Private Practice
Safford, Arizona

with 81 *illustrations*

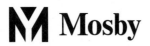 Mosby

St. Louis Baltimore Boston Chicago London Madrid Philadelphia Sydney Toronto

ΝΑ Mosby

Publisher: George Stamathis
Editor-in-Chief: Don Ladig
Executive Editor: Linda L. Duncan
Developmental Editor: Melba Steube
Project Manager: Linda Clarke
Production Editor: Allan S. Kleinberg
Manufacturing Supervisor: Kathy Grone

Printed in the United States of America

Mosby–Year Book, Inc.
11830 Westline Industrial Drive
St. Louis, Missouri 63146

Library of Congress Cataloging in Publication Data

Decision making in dental treatment planning / [edited by] Walter B.
  Hall, W. Eugene Roberts, Eugene E. LaBarre; artwork by Eric Curtis.
       p.   cm.
    Includes bibliographical references and index.
    ISBN 1–55664–241–5
    1. Dental therapeutics—Planning.   2. Dental therapeutics—
  –Decision making.   I. Hall, Walter B.   II. Roberts W. Eugene.
  III. LaBarre, Eugene E.
    [DNLM: 1. Dental Care.   2. Patient Care Planning.   WU 29 D294
  1994]
  RK318.D43   1994
  617.6—dc20
  DNLM/DLC
  for Library of Congress   93–2074
                                                                  CIP

94 95 96 97 98 CL/MVY 9 8 7 6 5 4 3 2

CONTRIBUTORS

GORDON R. ARBUCKLE, D.D.S., M.S.D.

Assistant Professor, Orthodontics
University of Indiana, School of Dentistry
Indianapolis, Indiana

JAMES J. BALDWIN, D.D.S., M.S.D.

Assistant Professor, Orthodontics
University of Indiana, School of Dentistry
Indianapolis, Indiana

BURTON E. BECKER, D.D.S.

Private Practice, Periodontics
Tucson, Arizona

WILLIAM BECKER, D.D.S., M.S.D.

Private Practice, Periodontics
Tucson, Arizona

W. PAUL BROWN, D.D.S.

Assistant Professor, Endodontics
University of the Pacific, School of Dentistry
San Francisco, California

GRETCHEN J. BRUCE, B.A., B.S., D.D.S.

Assistant Professor, Periodontics
University of the Pacific, School of Dentistry
San Francisco, California

JORDI J. CAMBRA, M.D., D.D.S.

Privte Practice, Periodontics
Barcelona, Spain

DAVID B. CLARK, D.D.S., M.S.D.

Assistant Professor, Orthodontics
University of Indiana, School of Dentistry
Indianapolis, Indiana

CARLO CLAUSER, M.D.

Private Practice, Maxillo-Facial Surgery
Florence, Italy

PIERPAOLO CORTELLINI, M.D., D.D.S.

Periodontology
University of Siena, Dental School
Siena, Italy

JAIME DELRIO-HIGHSMITH, M.D., D.D.S.

University of Madrid, Faculty of Dentistry
Madrid, Spain

HIPOLITO FABRA-CAMPOS, M.D., D.D.S.

Private Practice, Endodontics
Valencia, Spain

TIMOTHY F. GERACI, D.D.S., M.S.D.

Privte Practice, Endodontics
Oakland, California

JAMIE A. GIL-LOZANO, M.D., D.D.S.

Associate Professor and Chairman, Prosthodontics
University of The Basque Country,
Faculty of Medicine and Dentistry
Bilbao, Spain

ALAN H. GLUSKIN, A.B., D.D.S.

Associate Professor and Chair, Endodontics
University of the Pacific, School of Dentistry
San Francisco, California

WILLIAM W. Y. GOON, D.D.S.

Associate Professor of Endodontics
University of the Pacific, School of Dentistry
San Francisco, California

GENE A. GOWDEY, B.A., D.D.S.

Assistant Professor, Diagnostic Sciences
University of the Pacific, School of Dentistry
San Francisco, California

WALTER B. HALL, A.B., D.D.S., M.S.D.

Professor and Chair, Periodontics
University of the Pacific, School of Dentistry
San Francisco, California

WILLIAM F. HOHLT, D.D.S.

Assistant Professor, Orthodontics
University of Indiana, School of Dentistry
Indianapolis, Indiana

JOHN KWAN, D.D.S.

Private Practice, Periodontics
Oakland, California

EUGENE E. LABARRE, B.A., D.M.D., M.S.

Associate Professor and Chair, Removable Prosthodontics
University of the Pacific, School of Dentistry
San Francisco, California

CASIMIR LEKNIUS, D.D.S., M.S.

Assistant Professor, Fixed Prosthodontics
University of the Pacific, School of Dentistry
San Francisco, California

WILLIAM P. LUNDERGAN, D.D.S.

Associate Professor, Periodontics
University of the Pacific, School of Dentistry
San Francisco, California

KATHY I. MUELLER, D.D.S., D.M.D.

Assistant Professor, Fixed Prosthodontics
University of the Pacific, School of Dentistry
San Francisco, California

NEAL MURPHY, D.D.S., M.S.

Lecturer, Orthodontics and Periodontics
University of California, Los Angeles
School of Dentistry
Los Angeles, California

I. E. NAERT, D.D.S.

Lecturer, Prosthetic Dentistry
Catholic University of Leuven
School of Dentistry
Leuven, Belgium

ARUN NAYYAR, D.M.S., M.S.

Associate Professor and Director, Fixed Prosthodontics
Medical College of Georgia
School of Dentistry
Augusta, Georgia

MICHAEL NEWMAN, B.A., D.D.S.

Professor, Periodontics
University of California, Los Angeles
School of Dentistry
Los Angeles, California

JOAN PI URGELL, M.D., D.D.S.

Private Practice, Implantology
Barcelona and Granollers, Spain

GIOVAN PAOLO PINI-PRATO, M.D., D.D.S.

Professor and Chairman, Periodontology
University of Siena, School of Dentistry
Siena, Italy

W. EUGENE ROBERTS, D.D.S., PH.D.

Professor and Chairman, Orthodontics
University of Indiana, School of Dentistry
Indianapolis, Indiana

JOSE MANUEL ROIG-GARCIA, M.D., D.D.S.

Private Practice, Endodontics
Valencia, Spain

DAVID L. ROTHMAN, B.A., D.D.S.

Associate Professor and Chair, Pediatric Dentistry
University of the Pacific, School of Dentistry
San Francisco, California

MARIANO SANZ, M.D., D.D.S.

Associate Professor and Chairman, Periodontology
University of Madrid, School of Dentistry
Madrid, Spain

JAIME A. SAN MARTIN

Interim Professor, Prosthodontics
University of the Basque Country,
Faculty of Medicine and Dentistry
Bilbao, Spain

ROBERT SARKA, B.S., D.D.S., M.S.

Associate Professor, Removable Prosthodontics
University of the Pacific, School of Dentistry
San Francisco, California

HUGO SCHMIDT III, D.D.S.

Assistant Professor, Removable Prosthodontics
University of the Pacific, School of Dentistry
San Francisco, California

JOSEPH H. SCHULZ, D.D.S.

Associate Professor, Endodontics
University of the Pacific, School of Dentistry
San Francisco, California

ALBERTO SICILIA, M.D., D.D.S.

Associate Professor, Periodontology
University of Oviedo, School of Dentistry
Oviedo, Spain

E. ROBERT STULTZ, Jr., D.M.D., M.S.

Assistant Professor, Periodontics
University of the Pacific, School of Dentistry
San Francisco, California

CHARLES F. SUMNER III, D.D.S., J.D.

Associate Professor, Periodontics
University of the Pacific, School of Dentistry
San Francisco, California

MARK D. SUTTER, B.S., D.D.S.

Assistant Professor, Periodontics
University of the Pacific, School of Dentistry
San Francisco, California

JOSE MARIA TEJERINA, M.D., D.D.S.

Professor and Chairman, Periodontology
University of Oviedo, School of Dentistry
Oviedo, Spain

CHI TRAN, D.D.S.

Assistant Professor, Fixed Prosthodontics
University of the Pacific, School of Dentistry
San Francisco, California

GALEN W. WAGNILD, D.D.S., M.S.

Associate Professor, Restorative Dentistry
University of California, School of Dentistry
San Francisco, California

BORJA ZABELEGUI, M.D., D.D.S.

Private Practice, Endodontics
Bilbao, Spain

JON ZABELEGUI, M.D., D.D.S.

Private Practice, Endodontics
Bilbao, Spain

MARK ZABLOTSKY, B.S., D.D.S.

Assistant Professor, Periodontics
University of Pacific, School of Dentistry
San Francisco, California

For their love, support, and understanding
during the preparation of this text,
we dedicate it to our wives and children:
Francella, Scott, and Greg Hall
Cheryl, Carrie, and Jeffery Roberts
Denise, Elizabeth, Andrew, and Suzanne LaBarre

PREFACE

Decision Making in Dental Treatment Planning is an effort to illustrate the thought processes of dentists in several of the clinical specialties when their specific aspect of care is involved in complex dental cases. It is a logical progression from an earlier text, *Decision Making in Periodontology*, wherein the decision making process in only one field was presented. In complex cases, the periodontist would not attempt to dictate the whole treatment plan. He would correlate his treatment plan with what those performing other aspects of care believed would work best; thus, in complex case treatment planning, the difficulties which a general dentist tackles daily confront the specialist but in an even more complex way. He must work with the decisions made by others and sequence his treatment to achieve an end result agreed upon by the patient and all of those treating. The general dentist often must make all of these decisions himself, sometimes a daunting task, and one in which he should know when to seek help from the appropriate specialists.

This text presents decision making for treatment planning complex, interdisciplinary cases as viewed by specialists in Periodontics, Endodontics, Orthodontics, Prosthodontics, and Pediatric Dentistry. Conflicting viewpoints between specialists will be evident to the reader. As he must do in practice, the individual dentist must resolve these differences in order to present treatment plan options to the patient. This text should be helpful to the dentist in comprehending how various experts "think" in their decision making processes. Each reader can weigh the merits of any conflicting approaches presented by various contributors and arrive at his own conclusions while better understanding how others may arrive at different conclusions.

As new treatment approaches are presented and validated in practice, decision making in treatment planning changes, often becoming more complex. In the last decade, implants and guided tissue regeneration have greatly altered the options available for treatment. Some older approaches to treatment can be replaced with far superior new ones (e.g., rather than extracting or maintaining teeth which in the past were labeled "hopeless," such as second molars with large three-walled distal defects, guided tissue regeneration can totally change their prognosis with a high level of predictability). The cost of some newer approaches can be very high (e.g., implants) or can greatly reduce the cost of options such as bridge construction (e.g., regenerating a severe Class II furca defect on an endangered tooth rather than extracting it and placing a bridge). Patients have a right to know the pros and cons of each these approaches. The dentist must be able to verbalize the deductive process he employs to arrive at appropriate treatment options. This text should be helpful to the practicing dentist in improving his skills in this aspect of daily practice. For the student, it should be helpful in teaching him how he will use what he has learned.

Our thanks go to Brian Decker who conceived the "decision making" concept of medical and dental texts, to the editors at Mosby, Allan Kleinberg and Melba Steube, for their expertise and patience, to Belle Endzweig and Pagan Marshall for typing the manuscript, to our many contributors who made the text possible, to Eric Curtis for his illustrations, and to our families for their support and encouragement in preparing this book.

Walter B. Hall
W. Eugene Roberts
Eugene E. LaBarre

CONTENTS

ORTHODONTICS

PROSTHODONTICS

PEDIATRIC DENTISTRY

INTRODUCTION

Each two- to four-page chapter in this text consists of an algorithm or decision tree, which appears on the right-hand page, and a brief explanatory text with illustrations and references, which appears on the left-hand page. The decision tree is the focus of each chapter and should be studied first in detail. The letters on the decision tree refer the reader to the text, which provides a brief explanation of the basis for each decision. Boxes have been used on the decision tree to indicate invasive procedures or the use of drugs. Dotted-line boxes indicate the nature of major decisions that must be made. A combination of line drawings and half tones were selected to clarify the text. Cross references have been inserted to avoid repeating information given in other chapters. References that are readily available to the practitioner have been selected.

For reader convenience, the text has been divided into sections from the following specialty areas: Periodontics, Endodontics, Orthodontics, Prosthodontics, and Pedodontics. An index is included to facilitate the location of specific information.

The decisions outlined here relate to typical situations. Unusual cases may require the clinician to consider alternatives; however, in every case, the clinician must consider all aspects of an individual patient's data. The algorithms presented here are not meant to represent a rigid guideline for thinking but rather a skeleton to be fleshed out by additional factors in each individual patient's case. Because different specialty areas may view a problem in different ways, the reader must evaluate each of these differing views to arrive at the appropriate treatment plan for each individual patient.

PERIODONTICS

Walter B. Hall, Editor

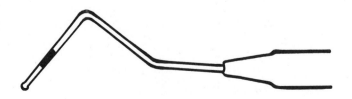

SEQUENCE OF PERIODONTAL TREATMENT

Walter B. Hall

When a patient with a complex dental problem presents for treatment, he must articulate his concept of the problem and his goals in seeking care. His medical, dental, and oral hygiene history must be evaluated. A full periodontal examination and radiographic evaluation must be performed. The first treatment planning decisions the dentist makes relate to an assessment of the periodontal aspects of the case upon which the restoration is to be based.

A. If no significant periodontal problem is present, he would continue to develop the overall treatment plan.

B. If a significant periodontal problem exists, he first must determine whether any aspects of the problem are acute (symptomatic) in nature. Acute problems require immediate attention that might preclude further treatment planning. The acute problems may be periodontal or endodontic in nature or both (combined). Such acute problems as human immunodeficiency virus HIV-gingivitis, HIV-periodontitis, necrotizing ulcerative gingivitis/necrotizing ulcerative periodontitis, herpetic gingivostomatitis, periodontal abscess, cracked tooth syndrome, or temporomandibular pain-dysfunction syndrome require immediate attention. The dentist must decide whether to treat the problem or refer the patient to a specialist promptly.

C. If no acute problem is present, the dentist must next make a difficult decision. Is he capable of performing the needed care or is referral to a specialist necessary (see p 6)? If his decision is to refer the patient, he should do so promptly. If the patient refuses the referral, the dentist must decide whether to treat a case he feels unequipped to handle well (which is unwise but sometimes necessary) or to refuse to accept the person as his patient.

D. If the dentist decides that he can perform the necessary periodontal care within acceptable standards, he must decide whether to proceed with the periodontal treatment or to obtain the aid of other appropriate specialists whose participation in the treatment may be needed. Most specialists want to be involved in the development of an overall treatment plan from the start so that they do not find themselves committed to a treatment-plan-in-progress in a case that they would have preferred to treat differently. If the dentist feels that he needs the participation of a specialist, he should seek it before beginning any nonemergency treatment.

References

Carranza FA. Clinical periodontology. 7th ed. Philadelphia: WB Saunders, 1990:552.

Corn H, Marks MH. Strategic extractions in periodontal therapy. Dent Clin North Am 1969; 13:817.

Grant DA, Stern IB, Listgarten MA. Periodontics. 6th ed. St Louis: Mosby, 1988:598.

Schluger S, Yuodelis R, Page RC, Johnson RH. Periodontal diseases. 2nd ed. Philadelphia: Lea & Febiger, 1990:331.

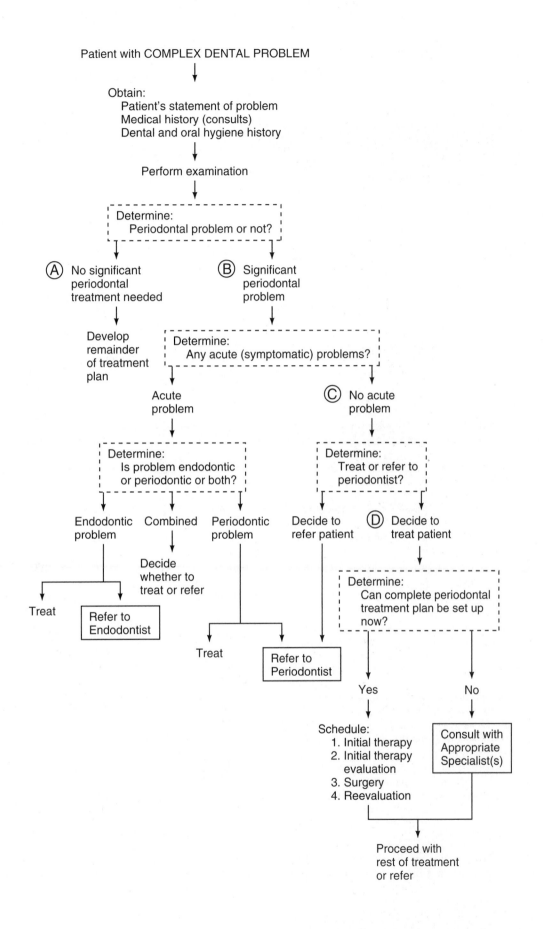

Patient with COMPLEX DENTAL PROBLEM

Obtain:
    Patient's statement of problem
    Medical history (consults)
    Dental and oral hygiene history

Perform examination

Determine:
    Periodontal problem or not?

Ⓐ No significant periodontal treatment needed

Ⓑ Significant periodontal problem

Develop remainder of treatment plan

Determine:
    Any acute (symptomatic) problems?

Acute problem

Ⓒ No acute problem

Determine:
    Is problem endodontic or periodontic or both?

Determine:
    Treat or refer to periodontist?

Endodontic problem

Combined

Periodontic problem

Decide to refer patient

Ⓓ Decide to treat patient

Decide whether to treat or refer

Treat

Refer to Endodontist

Treat

Refer to Periodontist

Determine:
    Can complete periodontal treatment plan be set up now?

Yes

No

Schedule:
    1. Initial therapy
    2. Initial therapy evaluation
    3. Surgery
    4. Reevaluation

Consult with Appropriate Specialist(s)

Proceed with rest of treatment or refer

REFERRAL TO A PERIODONTIST

Walter B. Hall
Charles F. Sumner III

When there is a periodontal component to the treatment plan for a complex dental problem, several factors determine the need or desirability of referring the patient to a periodontist. Some dentists have mastered many aspects of periodontal care. A dentist must have a realistic concept of his own abilities and limitations. In some states a quasi-legal requirement for referral or offer of referral of complex cases has been developed. A patient with a complex problem needs to know that a specialist in periodontics exists and may be consulted. If a case has complexities involving multiple specialized areas, referral is especially desirable.

A. If there are no significant periodontal aspects in the treatment plan, referral is not necessary.[1]

B. If the treatment plan has a significant periodontal component, the dentist must decide whether he has the required skills to treat the periodontal problem or if better care could be provided by a specialist. If he does not have the skill, he must refer the patient to a periodontist or refuse to treat the case. General practitioners who have additional training may treat cases that are no longer in the earliest stages. Should the general dentist decide that the level of disease is within his ability to treat, however, he must still inform the patient that he, the patient, has a periodontal disease and what the extent of the disease is and that there are specialists in the treatment of this dental disease. To fail to so inform the patient would be to render care without a complete informed consent.[2,3]

C. If the dentist believes that he has the necessary skill to provide the periodontal treatment, he must decide whether referral would be in the best interest of the patient and/or whether he is required by practice concepts in his area to refer the case. He must make the patient aware that a specialist, the periodontist, is available for consultation. If the dentist feels that he can handle the case and if the patient selects treatment by the dentist, the dentist must decide whether to treat the case or to refuse to accept the person as his patient.

   The general practitioner who performs the necessary treatment with the patient's informed consent is bound to disclose to the patient if the treatment is not successful.[4] He must refer the patient to a specialist as soon as he becomes aware or should have become aware that the therapy he has initiated is not proving to be as effective as could be expected in the hands of a specialist.

D. If the dentist feels that he has the skill to manage the periodontal care, but that better care could be pro-vided by a periodontist, he must determine whether the patient is likely to accept the referral and can afford treatment by a specialist. If so, the patient should be referred. If not, the dentist may consider altering the plan so that he can manage it or refuse to accept the person as a patient. If the patient declines to be referred, the informed consent aspects of the discussion should be recorded in the chart.

A suggestion that the patient seek the care of a specialist is not enough. The practitioner is obliged to adequately inform the patient about the extent of the disease and the consequences if he fails to follow through with the referral.[5] The courts have found the dentist negligent in cases in which the patient has asserted that he was not made aware of the consequence of his failing to seek care. Thus it would be prudent to follow up on each of the referrals and not simply dismiss the patient who apparently has not taken the advice.

Some courts have held the referring dentist liable for not having warned the patient of the extent and type of care he would receive from the specialist.[6] However, in most instances it is the primary obligation of the specialist or a member of his staff to properly inform the patient and obtain a satisfactory informed consent.[7,8]

The patient is at a disadvantage should he need to rely only on his own resources to choose a specialist. Once having informed the patient of his need for special care, the dentist is obliged to assist the patient in making a prudent choice. Having fulfilled his obligation of referring the patient to a specialist whom he reasonably believes to be competent, the referring dentist is not held liable for the negligent acts of the specialist. An exception exists to this rule where there is a partnership or fiduciary relationship between the general practitioner and the specialist.

Having entered into a joint relationship with the patient in the care and treatment of that patient's periodontal disease, it is essential that some agreement be reached as to the responsibility of follow-up care once the case has been referred to a specialist. Furthermore, it is equally essential that the patient be made aware, and consents to, these plans.

Periodontal disease is more frequently controlled than cured. Having taken on the responsibility of care, both the general practitioner and the specialist must meet a community standard in all aspects of determining a diagnosis, planning treatment, and providing maintenance care. Both parties have a duty to inform the patient of their plans, their prognoses, and the consequences of not following the plans. They must also offer the patient an alternative plan, if available, describing its advantages and disadvantages. Only then can the patient make an informed decision and the dentist proceed with an informed consent.

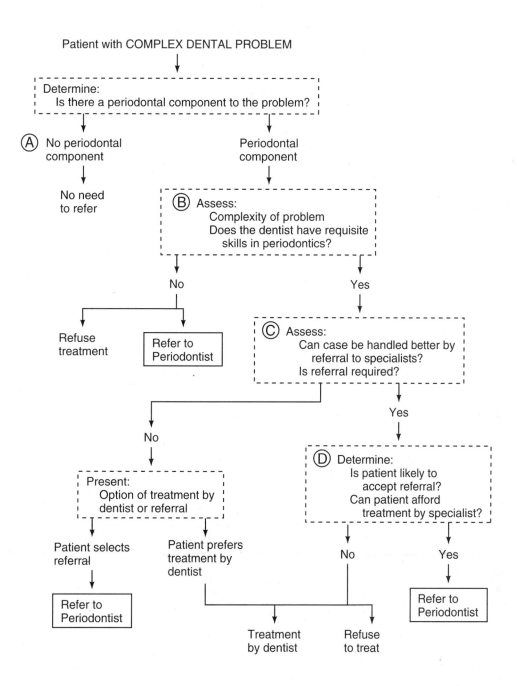

Patient with COMPLEX DENTAL PROBLEM

Determine:
Is there a periodontal component to the problem?

(A) No periodontal component

Periodontal component

No need to refer

(B) Assess:
Complexity of problem
Does the dentist have requisite skills in periodontics?

No

Yes

Refuse treatment

Refer to Periodontist

(C) Assess:
Can case be handled better by referral to specialists?
Is referral required?

No

Yes

Present:
Option of treatment by dentist or referral

(D) Determine:
Is patient likely to accept referral?
Can patient afford treatment by specialist?

Patient selects referral

Patient prefers treatment by dentist

No

Yes

Refer to Periodontist

Treatment by dentist

Refuse to treat

Refer to Periodontist

References

Grant DA, Stern IB, Listgarten MA. Periodontics. 6th ed. St Louis: Mosby, 1988:605.

Hall WB. Pure Mucogingival Problems. Berlin: Quintessence Publishing, 1984:169.

Zinman EJ. Common dental malpractice errors and preventive measures. J West Soc Periodont 1976; 23:149.

Legal References

1. Helling v. Carey, Wash. 519 P.2d 981 (1974).
2. Canterbury v. Spence, 464 F2d 772 (1972).
3. Cobbs v. Grant, 104 Cal Rptr. 505 (1972).
4. Baldor v. Roger, 81 S. Rptr 2d 660 (1955).
5. Moore v. Preventive Medicine Medical Group, Inc., 178 Cal. App.3d 728;223 Cal Rptr. 85 (1986).
6. Llera v. Wisner, 557 P.2d 805 (1976).
7. Mustacchio v. Parker, 535 So.2d 833 (La App.2Cir.1988).
8. Bulman v. Myers, D.D.S., 467 A.2d 1353 (Pa.Super.1983).
9. Kennedy v. Gaskell, 274 C.A. 2d 244;78 Cal. Rptr. 753 (1969).
10. Mayer v. Litow, 154 C.A. 2d 413;316 P.2d 351 (1957).
11. Wolfsmith v. Marsh, 51 C.2d, 832;337 P.2d 70 (1959).

HOPELESS TEETH

Walter B. Hall

When treating a patient with a complex dental problem, a decision regarding a tooth's prognosis as being "hopeless" is an important one early in treatment planning. Teeth with a hopeless prognosis should be considered for extraction (see p 10). The extent of loss of attachment, severity of furcation involvement, endodontic status, and restorability are the critical factors here.

Hopeless teeth are those that cannot be treated with reasonable expectations of eliminating or even controlling their dental problems. Such teeth are not always extracted; in some situations they may be maintained, occasionally for years, while fully recognizing that no means of treating them or stopping their loss of attachment exist. For example, a patient may have lost 50% or more of the attachment on his remaining teeth. Pocket elimination surgery might be ruled out on the basis that there would no longer be adequate support to keep the teeth with any reasonable degree of comfort or function. A Widman flap might be employed to debride the area once fully, but neither the patient nor the dentist could expect to control the disease process with root planing even with use of antibiotics. If the patient demanded, teeth might be maintained for some time before abscesses and pain would necessitate their removal. Patients should be aware of the hopelessness of the prognosis, the risks of abscesses, and the possible danger to general health; therefore, the concept of "hopelessness" should be explained fully when such a prognosis is used, so that the patient not only understands all the attendant risks of keeping such teeth but also is fully informed in the legal sense (see p 6). In the 1980s many teeth previously regarded as "hopeless" became salvageable by means of guided tissue regeneration pioneered in Sweden. Badly involved class II furcation involvements, large three-walled infrabony defects, and osseous craters, which were all nontreatable, are now predictably treatable. Significant numbers of formerly hopeless teeth can be saved by this means today. Further advances with this approach (e.g., guided tissue regeneration [GTR] for class III furcations) are imminent, which will further decrease the number of problems that will be regarded as "hopeless."

A. Loss of attachment is the most common reason for a prognosis of "hopelessness" for a tooth. When a tooth has lost more than 50% of its attachment, its potential usefulness and ability to be maintained often are related to the status of other teeth in the mouth; if other teeth with adequate support remain, it may be splinted and saved. If not, its long-term prognosis usually is viewed as hopeless. If a tooth has lost less than 50% of its attachment but has a pocket that approaches its apex (or apices), its prognosis is greatly affected by the character of the adjacent osseous lesion. If the deep pocket is within a narrow, three-walled defect, treatment with a bone regeneration procedure could greatly improve its prognosis (see p 54). If there is no

three-walled defect but the tooth is endodontically involved, endodontic treatment could improve its prognosis greatly. If no endodontic lesion is present and neither bone regeneration nor endodontics is to be performed, the prognosis is hopeless.

Some teeth continue to be regarded as hopeless because they are not restorable, because they are malposed to an extent not correctable orthodontically, or because of vertical or spiral cracks extending apically down their roots.

B. If the tooth is a molar with a class III furcation involvement (see p 60), its endodontic status should be determined. If endodontic therapy is needed and can be performed, the prognosis for the tooth is greatly improved. If not, the possibilities of improving the molar's prognosis depend on the possibility of root amputation or hemisection being employed to eliminate the furcation involvement and to create a maintainable situation on the remaining portion of the tooth. If this could not be done (because of root form or fusion), the prognosis is hopeless.

The endodontic health of a severely periodontally involved tooth should be assessed next. If a tooth is endodontically involved but not endodontically treatable (e.g., because of calcified canals, roots too crooked to be obturated, severely internally or externally reverted or perforated), it should be regarded as hopeless.

C. If the tooth is nonrestorable because of the caries or fracture status of its remaining portion, it should be viewed as hopeless even if it is maintained and periodontal treatment continues. If the tooth is not endodontically involved or is endodontically treatable, the next step is to determine whether it is treatable periodontally.

D. If a periodontally involved tooth is badly malposed, it still might be a useful tooth if it can be treated orthodontically. If a tooth can be moved into, or out of, certain types of osseous defects (see p 24), its prognosis may be greatly improved. If not, its prognosis may be hopeless regardless of the severity of the periodontal problem.

Usually, a tooth with less than 50% loss of attachment (LOA) is treatable by frequent root planing (see p 30) or with mucogingival osseous surgery (see p 34). Teeth with more than 50% LOA usually require more extensive treatment if they are to be saved.

E. Cracked tooth problems can make a tooth's prognosis hopeless. If "cracked tooth syndrome" exists and the symptoms are bothersome to the patient, the tooth may have to be removed if the crack extends vertically down the root. If the crack is essentially in the crown,

Patient with a PERIODONTALLY INVOLVED TOOTH

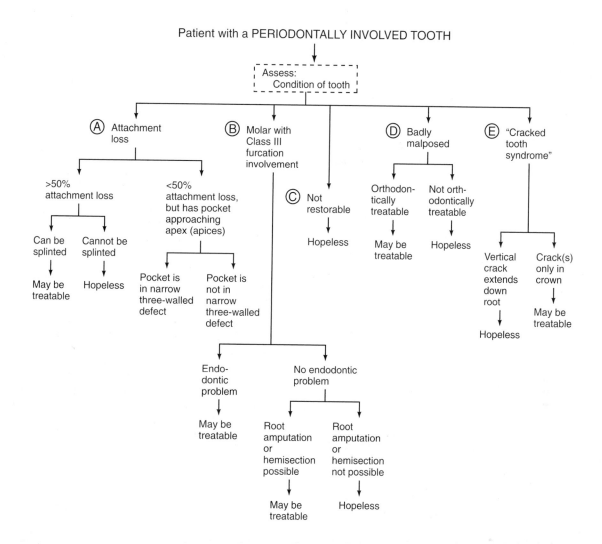

placing a restorative crown may control the symptoms, restrict further crack spreading, and improve the prognosis for the tooth. Vertical cracks in the root of the tooth are not treatable, however, and the prognosis is hopeless.

Some teeth with more than 50% LOA may be salvaged by GTR with highly predictable success. Teeth with class II or III furcation involvement (see p 58) may be treatable. Most class II furcation involvements with greater than 3 mm of horizontal loss into the furca but not "through and through" problems are good candidates for GTR. Teeth with class III furcation involvements may be treatable by GTR in the future, but root amputation, hemisection, or a tunnel operation have more predictable results today. If the roots are fused too far apically or are apically fused, such approaches cannot be used and the tooth should be regarded as hopeless. Teeth with three-walled defects, even of severe depth, routinely regenerate if the defect is narrow, that is, no more than 1 mm horizontally from tooth to crest of bone. If the three-walled defect is wider, GTR can be expected to be routinely successful. Teeth with a two-walled infrabony crater can be successfully treated by GTR unless their roots are less than 2 mm apart or the proximal furcas are too severely involved to be instru-

mented as a result of restricted access in which case they should be regarded as hopeless unless root amputation, hemisection, or extraction of one of the involved teeth makes the defect on the remaining one treatable. A tooth with more than 50% LOA that is not amenable to GTR can still be maintained if it can be splinted to other less involved teeth. If such splinting is not possible, the tooth should be regarded as hopeless.

References

Beube EC. Correlation of degree of alveolar bone loss with other factors for determining the removal or retention of teeth. Dent Clin North Am 1969; 13:801.

Corn H, Marks MA. Strategic extractions in periodontal therapy. Dent Clin North Am 1969; 13:817.

Hall WB. Periodontal preparation of the mouth for restoration. Dent Clin North Am 1980; 24:195.

Saxe SR, Corman DK. Removal or retention of molar teeth: The problem of the furcation. Dent Clin North Am 1969; 13:783.

Schluger S, Yuodelis R, Page RC, Johnson RH. Periodontal Diseases. 2nd ed. Philadelphia: Lea & Febiger 1989:341.

PERIODONTAL REASONS TO EXTRACT A TOOTH

Walter B. Hall

When a patient with a complex dental problem has a periodontally badly involved tooth, one with 50% or more attachment loss, a decision must be made regarding the consequences of extracting the badly compromised tooth. Assessment of the value of the individual tooth to the overall treatment plan is the first step in deciding whether to extract or to attempt to retain the tooth.

A. If the tooth has no critical importance to the overall treatment plan, it should be extracted rather than maintained because it may compromise the success of the overall restorative plan.

B. If the tooth is critically important to the overall treatment plan, how the tooth would be used in that plan must be determined. If it will not be a critical abutment tooth, extraction may be the best option. If it might add to the likelihood of success of the treatment plan, its retention would not compromise other critical teeth, and a "strategic retreat" (should it fail) is planned, surgical treatment may be a valid approach. Maintenance with a poor-to-hopeless prognosis may be considered if its retention does not jeopardize the overall plan or the chances for retaining it for a significant portion of the patient's remaining life seem good.

C. If the tooth is a critical abutment, the chances of treating it periodontally with reasonable likelihood of retaining it for a significant period should be assessed. If the prognosis does not appear good, the possibility of replacing the tooth with an implant should be considered. If this cannot be done because of the anatomy of the area (see p 74) or because the patient is unable or unwilling to consider an implant, the tooth should be extracted and a removable prosthetic replacement plan devised.

D. If the tooth can be treated periodontally with a reasonable chance of maintaining it for a significant time, a decision should be made on the need for splinting prior to surgery. If needed, temporary or provisional splinting should be performed prior to surgery.

E. If splinting is not needed, the possibility of successful regeneration of lost attachment should be considered. If guided tissue regeneration can be performed predictably (see p 62), it should be done and its success evaluated after 6 months. If the tooth is not amenable to guided tissue regeneration, the tooth has a guarded prognosis and may be treated by other surgical means, the success of the procedure should be evaluated 2 to 6 months later. If treatment is successful in improving the prognosis of the tooth, restoration may be instituted at this time. If the tooth's prognosis does not merit its inclusion in the plan at the time of re-evaluation, it should be extracted and an alternative plan instituted.

References

Carranza FA. Clinical Periodontology. 7th ed. Philadelphia: WB Saunders, 1990:546.

Hall WB. Removal of third molars: A periodontal viewpoint. In: McDonald RE, Hart WC, Gilmore HW, Middleton RA, eds. Current Therapy in Dentistry. St Louis: Mosby, 1980:225.

Hall WB. Periodontal preparation of the mouth for restoration. Dent Clin North Am 1980; 24:195.

Laskin DM. Evaluation of the third molar problems. J Am Dent Assoc 1971; 82:824.

Schluger S, Yuodelis R, Page RC, Johnson RH. Periodontal Diseases. 2nd ed. Philadelphia: Lea & Febiger, 1989:346.

Sorrin S, Burman LR. A study of cases not amenable to periodontal therapy. J Am Dent Assoc 1944; 31:204.

Patient with COMPLEX DENTAL PROBLEM AND A PERIODONTALLY BADLY INVOLVED TOOTH

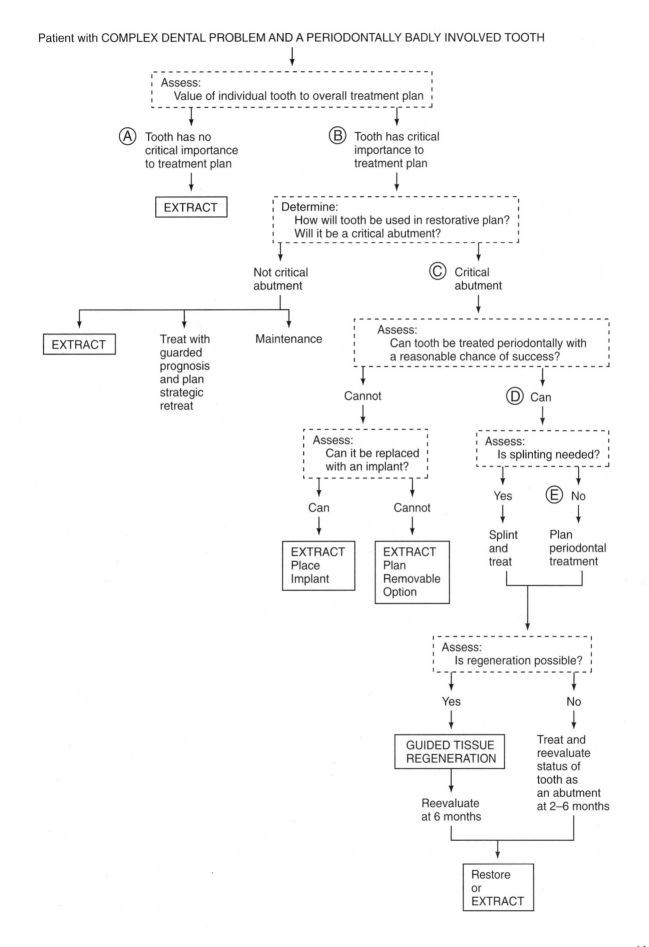

CRACKED TOOTH SYNDROME

Walter B. Hall

When a patient with a periodontal problem complains of pain localized to one tooth, especially if this is triggered by heavy function, the possibility that the tooth may be cracked should be investigated (Figs. 1, 2, and 3). If a tooth is cracked superficially, the symptoms may be controlled by crowning the tooth. Selective grinding may be helpful temporarily, but fractures tend to spread within teeth, making crowning the safest long-term solution for controlling these problems. A symptomatic crack may extend to involve the pulp. If the crack is deep already, endodontics may be helpful. If the tooth has been treated endodontically and now is symptomatic, the crack may be affecting the periodontal ligament. When a crack is contiguous with a deep pocket, the prognosis for the tooth is guarded at best, and therapy should be planned accordingly.

A. When a tooth with a periodontal pocket is painful, endodontic involvement must be ruled out before proceeding with any periodontal surgery. Whether or not the tooth is vital or nonvital on electrical pulp testing or to hot and cold, new periapical radiographs should be obtained and evaluated for evidence of periapical radiolucencies. The tooth should be evaluated visually and with a fiberoptic light source for cracks. The fiberoptic light stops at the plane of a crack where the light is defracted, and no glow of light extends to other parts of the tooth if the crack extends to the pulp. The tooth should be tapped and pressed in various directions against each cusp in an attempt to elicit the sharp, brief twinge of pain that is symptomatic of a cracked tooth.

B. If a symptomatic tooth tests vital, a radiograph may still suggest an endodontic problem. If no evidence (either visual or symptomatic) of a crack is elicited, selective grinding to minimize trauma should be employed. The tooth should be observed for several months to determine that symptoms have disappeared before any periodontal surgery is undertaken. If evidence of a crack is elicited, an orthodontic band should be cemented to minimize the likelihood of the crack's spreading. The dentist and patient should make a joint decision regarding whether to perform endodontic therapy promptly or to "wait and see" whether symptoms subside before any periodontal surgery is undertaken.

C. If a symptomatic tooth tests vital and has no evidence of periapical radiolucency, it should be examined for cracks or crack symptoms. If no evidence of a crack is elicited, selective grinding and observation for several months should be employed before any periodontal procedures are performed. If evidence of a crack is elicited, an orthodontic band or a stainless steel crown should be cemented to minimize fracture spread prior to any periodontal surgery.

Patient with POCKET DEPTH AND LOCALIZED PAIN OR TWINGES OF PAIN IN A TOOTH

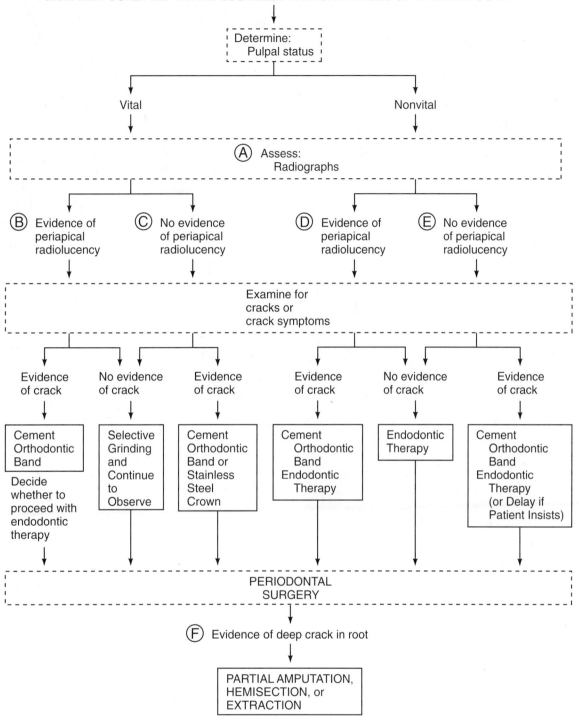

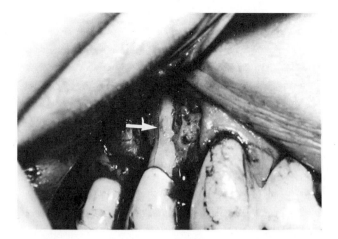

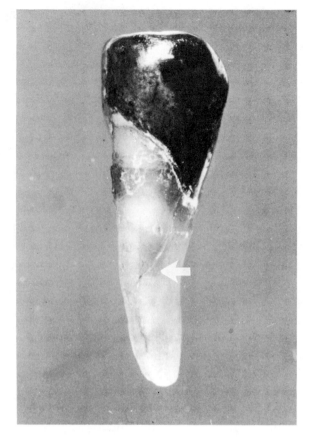

Figure 1. An endodontically treated first premolar with a vertical crack and a resulting deep periodontal defect.

Figure 3. Cracked tooth.

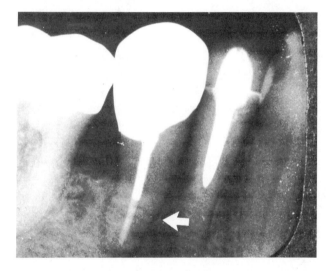

Figure 2. Vertical periodontal defect resulting from a cracked tooth.

D. If a symptomatic tooth tests nonvital, this may be confirmed by a radiographic periapical radiolucency. If so, the tooth should be examined for cracks. If no evidence of a crack is elicited, endodontic treatment should be completed promptly before any periodontal surgery is undertaken. If evidence of a crack is found, an orthodontic band should be cemented to its crown to minimize fracture spreading. The dentist and patient should make a joint decision to initiate endodontic promptly or to "wait and see." If symptoms do not subside, endodontics should be undertaken before any periodontal surgery. If symptoms subside, periodontal surgery could be undertaken with full recognition that an endodontic flare up could be precipitated, necessitating prompt endodontic treatment.

E. If a symptomatic tooth tests nonvital and radiographic evidence of a periapical radiolucency is not found, the tooth should be evaluated for evidence of a crack. If no evidence of a crack is elicited, the tooth should be treated endodontically before any periodontal surgery is performed. If evidence of a crack is elicited, an orthodontic band should be cemented to the crown and then endodontic treatment is performed before any periodontal surgery is undertaken.

F. When periodontal treatment is undertaken in any of these situations, a crack extending down the root where attachment has been lost may become visible. Once the area has been debrided, the fiberoptic light source may be employed to search for cracks. If a deep crack is found, the tooth may have to be extracted or possibly one root of a multirooted tooth may be amputated (in maxillary molars) or the tooth hemisected (in mandibular molars). If a patient elects not to have the tooth extracted, the dentist should carefully document the patient's choice and his advice that keeping the tooth is risky.

References

Cameron CE. The cracked tooth syndrome: Additional findings. J Am Dent Assoc 1976; 93:971.

Eahle WS, Maxwell EH, Braly BV. Fractures of posterior teeth in adults. J Am Dent Assoc 1986; 112:215.

Hiatt WH. Incomplete crown-root fracture. J Periodontal 1973; 44:369.

Maxwell EH, Braly BV. Incomplete tooth fracture: Prediction and prevention. Calif Dent Assoc J 1977; 5:51.

Ritchey B, Mendenhall R, Orban B. Pulpitis resulting from incomplete tooth fracture. Oral Surg Oral Med Oral Pathol 1957; 10:665.

IMPACTED THIRD MOLARS

Walter B. Hall

When a patient with a complex dental problem has impacted third molars present, his treatment plan should include decisions regarding the retention or extraction of those teeth. For younger patients the rationale for extracting such problem or potential problem teeth is stronger. Depending on the age of the older patient and estimates of his life expectancy, if the impacted third molars have not been causing problems, a decision to extract them is more difficult. If their retention would jeopardize the overall treatment plan, however, they should be removed.

Impacted third molars often create serious periodontal problems in adjacent teeth, or they become involved with periodontal problems on adjacent teeth as they develop. Early extraction of developing third molars may prevent some of these problems from occurring; however, patients are often hesitant regarding treatment of potential problems that are not symptomatic. As an impacted third molar develops, it may grow increasingly closer to the second molar root (Fig. 1). Once it is close, removal of the third molar may result in pocket depth distal to the second molar. Such surgically related pockets usually are accompanied by a three-walled residual osseous defect. If the defect is narrow, it may be amenable to a bone regeneration procedure. The decision as to residual pocket depth and the possibility of bone regeneration should be delayed for 6 months or more following the extraction.

A. If the impacted third molar is not close to the root of the second molar and the third molar is fully formed, the decision to retain or extract it is not a periodontal one. Likewise, if the third molar is still developing and it appears unlikely that it will ever come close to the root of the second molar, the decision to retain or extract is not a periodontal one. If further development of the third molar is unlikely to result in its crown's approaching the second molar root, however, the prompt extraction of the third molar is desirable periodontally.

B. If the impacted third molar already is close to, or is touching, the root of the second molar, the existing periodontal status of the second molar influences decisions regarding the third molar.

C. If the second molar is not periodontally involved, prompt extraction of the third molar is desirable periodontally. Do not probe the distal surface of the second molar for 6 months. Then, if a pocket exists, and the osseous defect appears to be a three-walled one, its narrow portion would be amenable to osseous regeneration (see p 66). If the defect is wider (i.e., greater than 1 mm from root surface to the crest of the osseous defect), guided tissue regeneration (see p 66) would be the recommended method of regaining attachment. This approach should be used whether or not the distal furca is involved.

D. If the crown of an impacted third molar is close to a second molar root that is periodontally involved, the degree of bone loss on the second molar influences treatment planning. If the bone loss is early to moderate and the third molar could erupt to replace the second molar, consider extraction of the second molar. If a probe placed in the distal defect on the second molar can touch the third molar, guided tissue regeneration can be used as a means of regaining lost attachment on the second molar; alternatively, extraction of both molars is a better means of fulfilling the overall treatment plan goals. If the crown of the third molar cannot be touched, the extraction may be delayed but is still periodontally desirable. If the third molar is unlikely to erupt to adequately replace the second molar, extract the third molar promptly if its crown can be touched or later if it cannot be touched. If the second molar has advanced bone loss but the third molar could erupt into adequate position to replace it, extract the second molar promptly. If the third molar is unlikely to erupt to replace the second molar, another option available to the patient would be extraction of the third molar and attempting to maintain the second (possibly with a modified Widman flap approach initially) or extraction of both molars (the sounder approach).

References

Ash MM, Costich ER, Hayward JR. Study of periodontal hazards or third molars. J Periodontal 1962; 33:209.

Ash MM. Third molars as periodontal problems. Dent Clin North Am 1964; 8:51.

Friedman JW. The case for preservation of third molars. J Calif Dent Assoc 1977; 5:50.

Hall WB. Removal of third molars: A periodontal viewpoint. In: McDonald RL, ed. Current Therapy in Dentistry. St Louis: Mosby, 1980:225.

Laskin DM. Indications and contraindications for removal of impacted third molars. Dent Clin North Am 1969; 13:919.

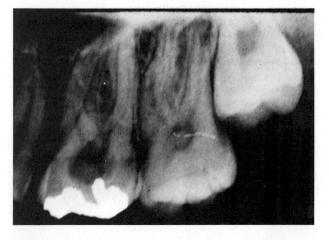

Figure 1. An impacted third molar appearing to contact the root of the adjacent second molar.

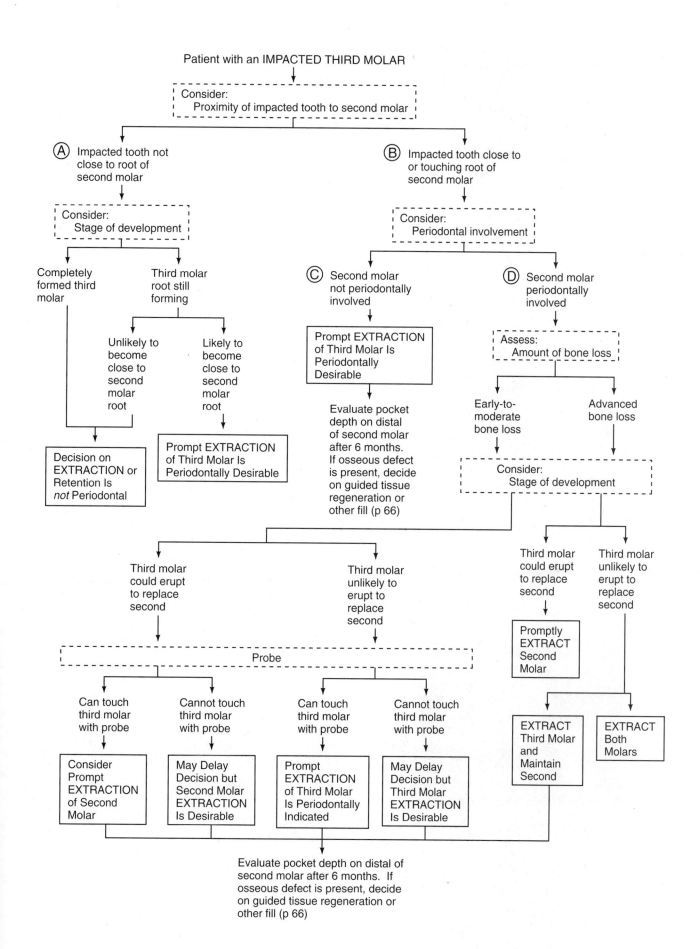

Patient with an IMPACTED THIRD MOLAR

Consider:
Proximity of impacted tooth to second molar

(A) Impacted tooth not close to root of second molar

Consider:
Stage of development

Completely formed third molar

Third molar root still forming

Unlikely to become close to second molar root

Likely to become close to second molar root

Decision on EXTRACTION or Retention Is *not* Periodontal

Prompt EXTRACTION of Third Molar Is Periodontally Desirable

(B) Impacted tooth close to or touching root of second molar

Consider:
Periodontal involvement

(C) Second molar not periodontally involved

Prompt EXTRACTION of Third Molar Is Periodontally Desirable

Evaluate pocket depth on distal of second molar after 6 months. If osseous defect is present, decide on guided tissue regeneration or other fill (p 66)

(D) Second molar periodontally involved

Assess:
Amount of bone loss

Early-to-moderate bone loss

Advanced bone loss

Consider:
Stage of development

Third molar could erupt to replace second

Third molar unlikely to erupt to replace second

Promptly EXTRACT Second Molar

EXTRACT Third Molar and Maintain Second

EXTRACT Both Molars

Third molar could erupt to replace second

Third molar unlikely to erupt to replace second

Probe

Can touch third molar with probe

Cannot touch third molar with probe

Can touch third molar with probe

Cannot touch third molar with probe

Consider Prompt EXTRACTION of Second Molar

May Delay Decision but Second Molar EXTRACTION Is Desirable

Prompt EXTRACTION of Third Molar Is Periodontally Indicated

May Delay Decision but Third Molar EXTRACTION Is Desirable

Evaluate pocket depth on distal of second molar after 6 months. If osseous defect is present, decide on guided tissue regeneration or other fill (p 66)

PARTIALLY ERUPTED THIRD MOLARS

Walter B. Hall

Partially erupted third molars present a unique set of periodontal problems. A partially erupted third molar has pocket depth at least to its cementoenamel junction. Although this is only a pseudo-pocket initially, it can lead to loss of attachment on the third molar and to pocket formation on the adjacent second molar. Extraction of the third molar before significant periodontal problems occur is desirable; if the third molar is impacted against the root of the second molar, however, a residual defect on the distal of the second molar is likely to occur following the extraction. This defect is more likely to occur than with fully impacted third molars, because insufficient gingiva to permit primary closure of the wound following third molar extraction is more likely to exist around partially erupted than around fully impacted teeth.

A. A third molar can be partially erupted but not in close proximity to the second molar (i.e., a vertical impaction in the ramus of the mandible). If the second molar is healthy or has had little bone loss, consider eventual extraction of the third molar. If the second molar has moderate-to-severe bone loss and the partially erupted third molar could be moved into good position following extraction of its neighbor, extraction of the second molar with orthodontic movement of the third molar (either moving it into its position or uprighting it for use as an abutment) is a good option.

B. If the partially erupted third molar is close to, or touching, the second molar (Fig. 1), other options apply. If the third molar is close to, or touching, the crown of the second molar only and the second molar has little or no bone loss, prompt extraction of the third molar is periodontally advisable before significant pocketing occurs distal to the second molar. If the second molar has moderate-to-advanced bone loss and the third molar has adequate remaining support, the second molar should be removed and the third molar moved orthodontically into its place, uprighted for use as an abutment, or replaced with an implant.

C. If the partially erupted third molar is close to, or touching, the root of the second molar, several possibilities exist. If the second molar has little or no bone loss and the third molar has little remaining support, prompt extraction of the third molar is indicated, with evaluation of the pocket status distal to the second molar no sooner than 6 months after the extraction. If a narrow three-walled defect (less than 1 mm horizontally from root to osseous crest) remains on the distal of the second molar, a Prichard-type bone fill (see p 64) is recommended. If the three-walled defect is wider, guided tissue regeneration (see p 66) should be employed whether or not the distal furca is involved. If the third molar has little or no bone loss and the second molar has moderate-to-advanced bone loss, the second molar could be extracted and the third molar moved orthodontically either into its place or uprighted to serve as an abutment. Alternatively, an implant could be employed to replace the second molar (see p 72). If both molars are badly involved, both should be extracted, as their relationship makes them prone to abscess formation because of the difficulty of cleaning by either the patient or the dentist. An implant could be employed to replace the extracted teeth.

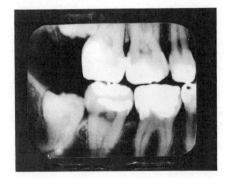

Figure 1. Partially erupted third molar appearing to be in close contact with the second molar.

References

Ash MM, Costich ER, Hayward JR. Study of periodontal hazards of third molars. J Periodontal 1962; 33:209.

Ash MM. Third molars as periodontal problems. Dent Clin North Am 1964; 8:51.

Braden BE. Deep distal pockets adjacent to terminal teeth. Dent Clin North Am 1969; 13:161.

Hall WB. Removal of third molars: A periodontal viewpoint. In: McDonald RL: Current Therapy in Dentistry. St Louis: Mosby, 1980:225.

Patient with a PARTIALLY ERUPTED THIRD MOLAR

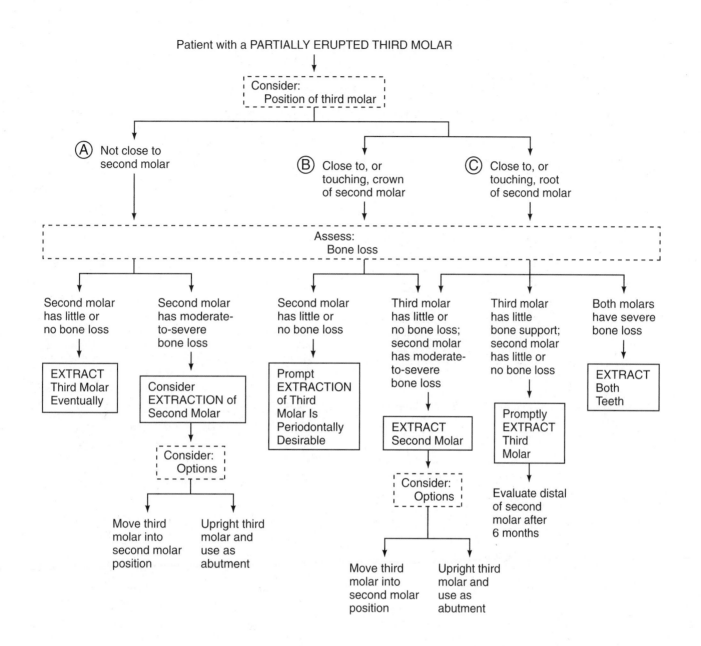

WHEN TO USE MICROBIAL TESTS FOR SPECIFIC PERIODONTAL PATHOGENS IN DIAGNOSIS AND TREATMENT PLANNING

Mariano Sanz
Michael Newman

The etiologic role of specific bacteria in certain periodontal diseases has been established in recent years. Although the majority of microorganisms found in deep periodontal pockets are part of the normal oral flora, a limited number of bacterial species is present only in periodontally diseased persons or carriers. A distinct group of subgingival pathogens has been associated with various types of periodontitis. The number of these species is elevated in active periodontitis lesions, has been reduced in or eliminated from successfully treated periodontitis sites, and has been detected in recurrent or refractory lesions. Therefore the detection of these potential periodontal pathogens or micro-organisms indicative of periodontitis, may have a role in the diagnosis and treatment of certain periodontal diseases.

In treating complex dental problems with a periodontal component, types of periodontitis that have severe or rapid onset or that do not respond well to initial therapy are significant determinants of treatment planning. Clinical measurements and radiographic evaluation and/or monitoring for progression of disease must be assessed to determine whether microbial tests can be useful. In many such cases these tests determine the direction of total treatment.

A. The age of the patient may determine the potential usefulness of microbial tests. Early onset periodontitis (e.g., juvenile periodontitis or mixed dentition periodontitis) is one such problem area. Identification of specific pathogens such as *Actinomycates actinomycetemcomitans, Porphyromonus gingivalis,* or *Prevotela intermedia* and their elimination following therapy are very useful in determining periodontal prognosis, which will govern the remaining dental treatment direction.

B. The severity of the problems may be assessed clinically and radiographically. Severe forms of periodontitis (deep pockets, mobile teeth) may be more definitively diagnosed with microbial testing. Upon diagnosis the appropriate antimicrobial therapy can be applied.

C. Less severe cases should be approached by conventional therapeutic means (e.g., root planing, plaque control). Refractory cases (i.e., those that do not respond adequately to these means) may benefit from microbial testing.

D. If the patient is an adult, slight-to-moderate problems are routinely managed with conventional therapy as are slowly progressive, more severe forms of periodontitis with no systemic involvement. If the lesion can be documented to be of rapid onset or if response to conventional therapy is not as expected, microbial testing often is useful. In refractory cases, the adequacy of the patients' plaque control efforts should be assessed before microbial testing is done. If the oral hygiene effort is poor, further plaque control therapy should be tried and its success reevaluated. If the plaque control is good and lesions remain refractory, microbial testing should be employed to determine the appropriate antimicrobial therapy.

References

Carranza FA. Clinical Periodontology. 7th ed. Philadelphia: WB Saunders, 1990:714.

Genco RJ, Zambon JJ, Christersson L. Use and interpretation of bacteriological assays in periodontal diseases. Oral Microbiol Immunol 1986; 1:73.

Lang NP, Brecx MC. Periodontal diagnosis in the 1990's. J Clin Periodontol 1991; 18:370.

Maiden JFJ, Carman RJ, Curtis MA, et al. Detection of high-risk groups and individuals for periodontal diseases: Laboratory markers based on the microbiological analysis of subgingival plaque. J Clin Periodontol 1990; 17:1.

Slots J, Rams TF. New views on periodontal microbiota in special patient categories. J Clin Periodontol 1991; 18:411.

Van Winkelhoff AJ, de Graaf J. Microbiology in the management of destructive periodontal disease. J Clin Periodontol 1991; 18:406.

A patient with a COMPLEX DENTAL PROBLEM WITH POCKET DEPTH, BONE LOSS, AND ATTACHMENT LOSS

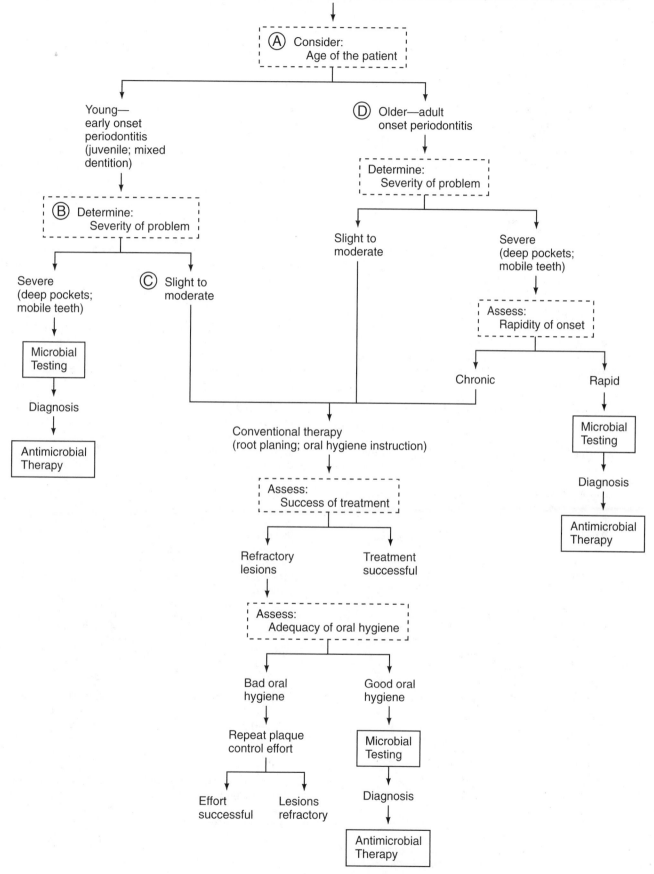

PERIODONTALLY COMPROMISED POTENTIAL ABUTMENT TEETH

Walter B. Hall

One of the most complex decisions that a dentist often must make involves the adequacy of periodontally involved teeth to function as abutments in a restorative treatment plan. The dentist must decide by weighing the advantages and disadvantages of each of the many factors involved. The patient must be informed of, and able to cope with, various degrees of uncertainty in such complex decisions and must be able to afford the cost of the whole treatment plan before it is initiated. If the patient elects not to proceed, the dentist must advise him of the probable consequences of this decision. Such complex situations require careful documentation.

A. The status of the attachment of the potential abutment tooth is very important. A tooth that has lost more than half of its attachment is a poor risk as an abutment. However, if that tooth has a narrow, three-walled osseous defect, it is a candidate for a bone regeneration procedure; in such cases the likelihood of success is reasonably sufficient to change the prognosis for the tooth. Moreover, in situations in which guided tissue regeneration has a strong probability of success (i.e., wide three-walled defects, deep class II furcations, many two-walled infrabony craters), a tooth that would be a poor abutment can be converted to one that may make a good-to-excellent abutment (see p 64). Otherwise, a tooth that has lost more than half of its support is unlikely to be a good abutment risk. If the tooth has moderate loss of attachment, it has a reasonable prognosis for successful use as an abutment. If it has little loss, it is a good candidate.

B. Root form is another important factor to assess. Several radiographs of the tooth can be used to conceptualize the form for the root (Fig. 1). Exploration of furcations

on a multirooted tooth can provide useful information on its potential cleansibility. Teeth with small or cone-shaped roots are poor abutments compared with teeth with large roots or multirooted teeth with flared roots. If a molar has a class II furca involvement of 3 mm or more horizontally but not a class III ("through and through") involvement, it is a good candidate for guided tissue regeneration and eventual use as an abutment (see p 62). If a molar has a "through and through" involvement, root amputation or hemisection may make its remaining parts useful as abutments if that approach is affordable to the patient (see p 58). A molar with minimal furcation involvement and flared roots is a good abutment candidate, however.

C. The status of the crown of the potential abutment is important too. If it is badly broken down, it is a poorer candidate than if it can be restored readily. Crown lengthening improves the potential restorability of some poorer status teeth (see pp 32 and 34).

D. The pulpal status affects the tooth's potential to be used as an abutment. If the tooth has been endodontically treated but requires further treatment (i.e., apicoectomy) or retreatment or appears to have a cracked root, its usefulness as an abutment depends on the likelihood of success of the additional treatment. If its root is cracked or it cannot be re-treated, it has no potential as an abutment. If the earlier endodontic procedure appears satisfactory, the tooth usually has good potential as an abutment. If the tooth has an untreated pulpal problem, its potential for use as an abutment depends on factors affecting the probability of successful endodontic treatment (i.e., accessibility of root canals, presence of pulp stones, internal resorption). If it is treatable, it has good potential as an abutment. A tooth with a healthy pulp, however, is almost always a better abutment candidate than an endodontically treated one, because endodontically treated teeth are more brittle and more susceptible to fractures.

E. The alignment of a tooth affects its usefulness as an abutment. A significant malposed tooth that cannot be orthodontically moved into good alignment has poor potential as an abutment. Some periodontally involved teeth are good candidates for orthodontic movement (see p 24) and can become fair-to-good candidates for use as abutments, but only at considerable cost to the patient both in time and money. A tooth already in normal alignment is usually a better candidate for use as an abutment.

F. The number of other abutment teeth and their periodontal status affect the potential usability of a tooth as an abutment. If other potential abutments are few and

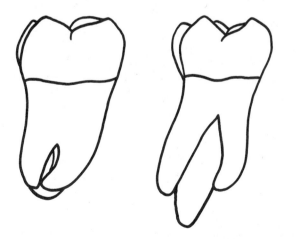

Figure 1. Molar teeth may have fused or spread roots. The spread type usually provides better support as an abutment for a restoration replacing a missing tooth.

Patient with PERIODONTALLY COMPROMISED POTENTIAL ABUTMENT TOOTH

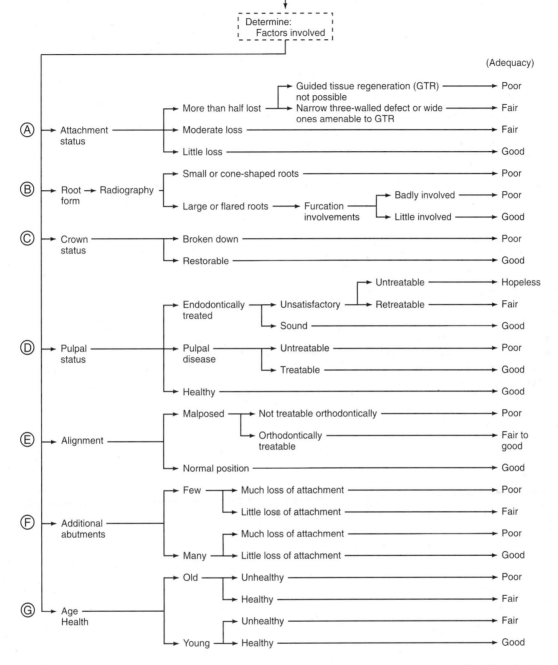

have much loss of attachment, the tooth in question is a poorer candidate for use as an abutment, because more is needed from it. If the other potential abutments are few but have little loss of attachment, the tooth in question is a better candidate. If there are many additional potential abutment teeth but all or most have significant loss of attachment, the potential use of the tooth in question is less. If the other potential abutments have lost little attachment, the tooth in question has better potential for use as an abutment.

G. Other factors (e.g., plaque-removal skills of the patient, regularity of dental care) must be weighed by the dentist and patient when determining the potential for a periodontally involved tooth to be used as an abutment. Age and health are essential factors, however. In one sense, older patients have poorer prog-

noses than younger ones in that their healing capabilities are likely to be lower; in another sense, older patients have better prognoses in that their teeth and dental work do not have to last as long on average. A potential abutment tooth that is periodontally compromised in an otherwise healthy patient usually has a better prognosis than one in an unhealthy mouth.

References

Grant DA, Stern IB, Listgarten MA. Periodontics. 6th ed. St Louis: Mosby, 1988:982, 1018.

Hall WB. Periodontal preparation of the mouth for restoration. Dent Clin North Am 1980; 24:195.

Schluger S, Yuodelis R, Page RC, Johnson RH. Periodontal Diseases. 2nd ed. Philadelphia: Lea & Febiger, 1990:341.

ORTHODONTICS AND PERIODONTAL NEEDS

Timothy F. Geraci

The goal of orthodontic tooth movement in an adult is to improve both the periodontal and restorative environments. The adult orthodontic candidate who presents with preexisting periodontal involvement requires a dentist with critical diagnostic skills, rigid periodontal therapeutic skills, and a knowledge of the biomechanical movement of teeth. An adult has a static orthodontic environment; the growth period has been completed and cannot be used in diagnostic planning. To make matters more complex, biomechanical intervention can either improve or worsen the periodontal status.

A. When the oral hygiene level is not acceptable, the patient should not undergo orthodontic therapy. The inflammatory lesion must be controlled during orthodontic movement; otherwise, the case could be compromised and/or teeth lost as a result of the orthodontics. Thorough root planing and root debridement are basic preorthodontic requirements if pathology is present. Surgical intervention may be required to ensure clean roots or reduction of nonmaintainable pocket depth. A periodontal abscess during the active orthodontic phase can be disastrous.

B. Interceptive mucogingival surgery should be performed in areas with potential problems. A compromised solution may result if the problem is not addressed until it is acute. Because of the position of the teeth in the alveolar housing, there may be a partial absence of bone over the facial or lingual root surface and a connective tissue attachment only. Failure to recognize this problem before treatment begins could result in severe root exposure during treatment and/or a tooth that is in a proper position but cannot be restored owing to lack of supporting bone.

C. The patient's root form and length are important with respect to postorthodontic suitability. Poor root form and length are absolute contraindications for orthodontic therapy. At the other end of the spectrum, teeth with long roots may not move easily or at all.

D. Teeth with preexisting furcation involvements of class II or more are poor candidates for orthodontic movement. The chances of an abscess or increased bone loss are too great. The involved tooth may be endodontically treated and the root or roots removed if the tooth is critical to the case. A tooth with class I furcation involvement requires the highest priority during orthodontic therapy, and it must be monitored and debrided constantly.

E. Patients who present with preexisting crepitus, muscle tenderness, excessive occlusal wear, restricted mandibular opening, mandibular deviation on opening and closing, or subluxation of the mandible are not good candidates for orthodontic tooth movement. Their conditions may not improve with orthodontic treatment and, in fact, may worsen. Their dental findings should be documented before beginning tooth movement.

F. If anterior teeth that have drifted to a facial position are going to be retracted to a functional position, sufficient overjet and overbite are required and an occlusal adjustment may be needed to place the mandible in a stable, retruded position. If a suitable overjet/overbite and stable occlusal position cannot be achieved, orthodontic movement cannot be successful. A diagnostic occlusal splint is indicated in preorthodontic therapy to determine if the above objectives can be achieved.

CASE PROGNOSIS DEPENDS ON IMPROVING THE PATIENT'S TOOTH POSITION

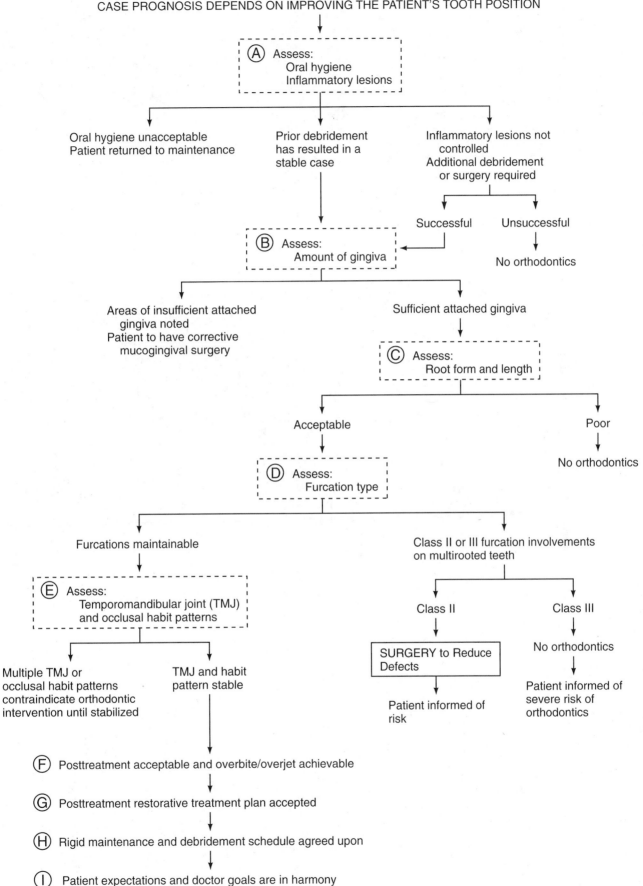

G. Before initiation of minor tooth movement procedures, the patient must be informed of the need to retain teeth in their new position via splinting or fixed bridgework and of the cost involved in restoring the case. If a tipped tooth is being placed in an upright position for fixed bridgework, occlusal reduction is required during treatment to gain space in an occlusal-apical direction for the tooth to move. Because of the "increase" in clinical crown during the uprighting and the reduction of the occlusal height to gain space, followed by crown preparation, a posterior tooth that has been uprighted may require an endodontic procedure (Figs. 1 and 2).

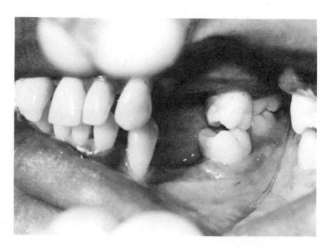

Figure 1. Preoperative view of a tilted molar with a mesial osseous defect prior to uprighting.

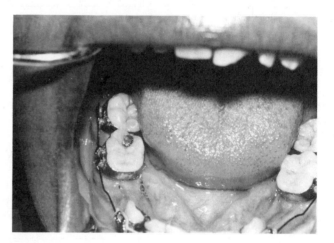

Figure 2. The same teeth with the orthodontic appliance in place to bring the tilted teeth upright.

H. Because orthodontic tooth movement involves a breakdown of bone where pressure is applied and deposition of bone in areas of application of tension, the osseous topography of an area changes as a result of tooth movement. Infrabony defects can be reduced by deposition of bone on the tension side of the root and positioning of the root into an infrabony defect on the pressure side of the root. During the active phase of movement the roots should be debrided and the soft tissue lining the pockets curettaged every 2 weeks. As stated above, the inflammatory lesion must be controlled during the active phase. Constant debridement of an area increases the chances for reducing an infrabony defect and for successful resolution of a case. Patients with more severe infrabony lesions should be placed on a strict 3 month periodontal maintenance program during their orthodontic therapy.

I. Finally, the patient should understand the objectives of minor tooth movement. The expectations of the patient and the goal of the doctor cannot be in conflict, and the dental objectives should be noted and discussed before treatment is initiated.

References

Lindhe J. Clinical Periodontology. 2nd ed. Copenhagen: Munksgaard, 1989:564.

Sadowsky C, BeCole E. Long-term effects of orthodontic treatment on periodontal health. Am J Orthod 1981; 80:156.

Zachrisson B, Alnaes L. Periodontal condition in orthodontically treated and untreated individuals. Part I. Angle Orthod 1973; 43:401.

Zachrisson B, Alnaes L. Periodontal conditions in orthodontically treated and untreated individuals. Part II. Angle Orthod 1974; 44:43.

SELECTIVE GRINDING VERSUS SPLINTING

Walter B. Hall

If a periodontal patient seeking treatment has loose teeth and would benefit if further trauma to them could be minimized, the dentist must decide whether to use selective grinding or splinting or a combination of the two.

A. The loose teeth may be localized or generalized. A localized problem offers more options than does a generalized one. A localized problem may be one of primary or secondary occlusal trauma. A generalized problem may be one mostly of primary, or mostly of secondary, occlusal trauma.

B. Localized loose teeth may have lost little or no bone support but still be mobile. Selective grinding should eliminate problems of localized, primary occlusal trauma.

C. Localized loose teeth could have lost a moderate-to-severe amount of bone. If most other teeth are sound (have little bone loss), selective grinding may reduce the loading to the loose teeth enough that trauma is minimized. If the adjacent teeth are sound and the loose tooth is moderately involved, splinting may be used to stabilize the loose tooth. If the loose tooth has lost substantial support, guided tissue regeneration (GTR) may be considered. If GTR is a predictable procedure on the severely involved tooth, it should be utilized (see p 54). If GTR is not possible or acceptable to the patient and the adjacent abutments are adequate, the compromised tooth should be extracted and replaced with a bridge rather than jeopardizing sound abutment teeth to maintain a tooth with a guarded to hopeless prognosis.

D. If most teeth are loose but have little or no bone loss, the problem is one of generalized primary occlusal trauma and can be managed with selective grinding. A night guard may also be required.

E. If most teeth have moderate-to-severe bone loss, generalized secondary occlusal trauma is the diagnosis. The possible use of GTR to change individual tooth prognosis should be assessed. Where practical, GTR should be employed along with temporary or provisional splinting before permanent splinting is done. In cases in which the amount of loss of support is less, splinting along with maintenance and/or surgery may be sufficient treatment. The age and financial means of the patient will influence the decision to proceed.

References

Carranza FM. Clinical Periodontology. 7th ed. Philadelphia: WB Saunders, 1990:422.

Nyman S, Lindhe J, Lundgren D. The role of occlusion for the stability of fixed bridges in patients with reduced periodontal support. J Clin Periodontol 1975:2253.

Ramfjord S, Ash MM. Occlusion. 3rd ed. Philadelphia: WB Saunders, 1983:384, 507.

Ringli HH. Splinting of teeth: An objective assessment. Helv Odontol Acta 1971; 15:129.

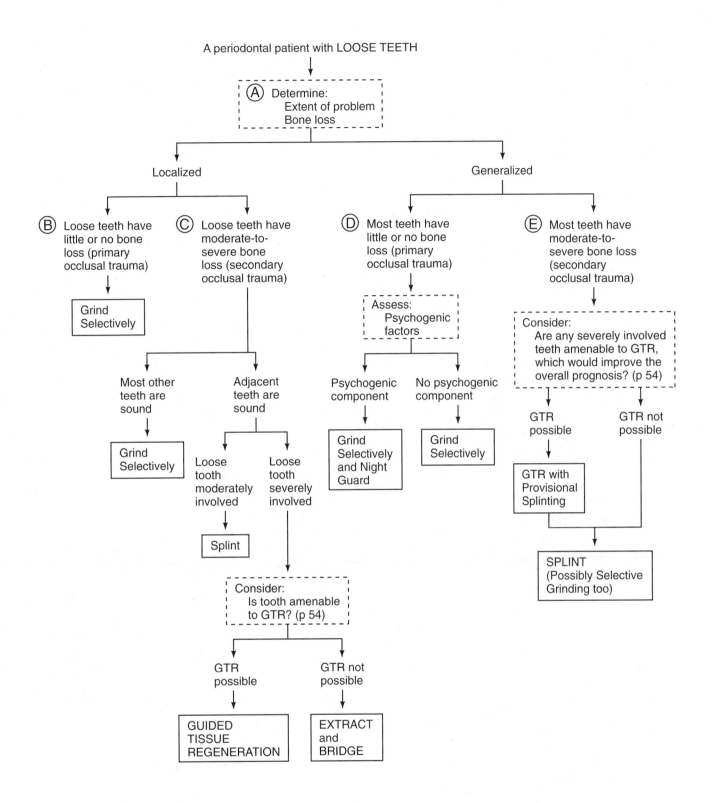

A periodontal patient with LOOSE TEETH

(A) Determine:
Extent of problem
Bone loss

Localized

Generalized

(B) Loose teeth have little or no bone loss (primary occlusal trauma)

Grind Selectively

(C) Loose teeth have moderate-to-severe bone loss (secondary occlusal trauma)

(D) Most teeth have little or no bone loss (primary occlusal trauma)

Assess:
Psychogenic factors

(E) Most teeth have moderate-to-severe bone loss (secondary occlusal trauma)

Consider:
Are any severely involved teeth amenable to GTR, which would improve the overall prognosis? (p 54)

Most other teeth are sound

Grind Selectively

Adjacent teeth are sound

Psychogenic component

Grind Selectively and Night Guard

No psychogenic component

Grind Selectively

GTR possible

GTR not possible

GTR with Provisional Splinting

SPLINT
(Possibly Selective Grinding too)

Loose tooth moderately involved

Splint

Loose tooth severely involved

Consider:
Is tooth amenable to GTR? (p 54)

GTR possible

GTR not possible

GUIDED TISSUE REGENERATION

EXTRACT and BRIDGE

SURGICAL THERAPY VERSUS MAINTENANCE

Timothy F. Geraci

A. The goal of periodontal therapy is to develop a stable state that the patient and the dentist can maintain with ease. The possibilities of attaining this goal are a determining factor in evaluating a case for surgery. If initial therapy (i.e., root planing and plaque control) has attained the goal of an easily maintainable case, maintenance planing and monitoring to determine continued stability may be all that is required. If a stable state cannot be attained or maintained with ease, surgical alteration may be useful in achieving this goal. The decision is made at the initial therapy evaluation, which should take place several weeks following completion of the initial treatment.

B. If the patient's general health is good, surgery may be considered. If he is seriously compromised (e.g., poorly controlled diabetes, high diastolic blood pressure), surgery may be contraindicated and the patient should be maintained as well as possible with frequent recall visits for instrumentation and oral hygiene efforts.

C. Plaque control by the patient is a key determining factor in deciding whether surgical therapy has merit or not. If the patient's plaque control on visible, accessible areas of the teeth is not good, mucogingival-osseous surgery would be as likely to compromise the case as to help it. Initial therapy should be repeated. If the patient's plaque control is good (or if there are overriding restorative demands), mucogingival-osseous surgery may be proposed.

D. Bleeding or suppuration on probing are indications that pocket areas that are inaccessible to plaque control measures at home continue to exhibit active disease. When bleeding or suppuration do not occur on probing, recall maintenance may be an adequate means of stabilizing the case. Restorative needs, however, could be an indication for surgery in spite of this stability. If plaque control on the visible, accessible parts of teeth is good but bleeding or suppuration occur on probing, surgery should be considered.

E. Surgery is indicated if it could make areas more accessible for plaque control and root planing without compromising support of potentially maintainable teeth or creating unacceptable esthetic situations owing to root exposure. If additional support can be gained by regenerative means, consideration of the surgical alternative should be encouraged vigorously. If these objectives cannot be attained surgically, recall maintenance would be the approach of choice. If they can be obtained, the surgical alternative should be proposed to the patient for his acceptance or rejection (see p 54).

References

Carranza F. Clinical periodontology. 7th ed. Philadelphia: WB Saunders, 1990:555.

Lindhe J. Textbook of clinical periodontology. 2nd ed. Copenhagen: Munksgaard, 1989:386.

Lindhe J, Nyman S. The effect of plaque control and surgical pocket elimination on the establishment and maintenance of periodontal health. A longitudinal study of periodontal therapy in cases of advanced periodontal disease. J Clin Periodontol 1985; 2:67.

Schluger S, Yuodelis R, Page RC, Johnson RH. Periodontal diseases. 2nd ed. Philadelphia: Lea & Febiger, 1990:461, 465.

Patient with RESIDUAL POCKET DEPTHS AT TIME OF INITIAL THERAPY EVALUATION

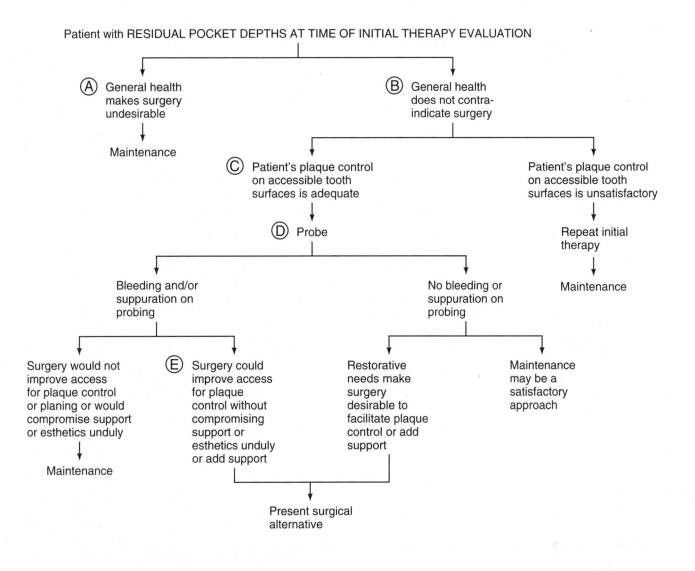

CROWN LENGTHENING

Gretchen J. Bruce

One of the challenges of restorative dentistry is the restoration of teeth with insufficient supragingival tooth height. Clinical situations that require a decision to restore or extract such a tooth are (1) short clinical crown, (2) root caries, (3) subgingival perforation, (4) fractures, (5) retrograde wear, and (6) altered passive eruption. When teeth are restored without regard to biologic principles, the periodontium may develop increased probing depths, problems with respect to plaque control, and a swollen cyanotic appearance.

"Biologic width" has been described as the space occupied by the junctional epithelium and connective tissue attachment coronal to the alveolar crest. This dimension is approximately 2.04 mm (Fig. 1). An additional millimeter representing the gingival crevice is combined with this figure to permit the establishment of an intracrevicular restorative margin. A minimum of 3 mm of sound tooth above the alveolar process is necessary when a restoration or fracture approaches the crest. Violation of the biologic width may result in inflammation and bone resorption. Surgical procedures such as gingivectomy, apically positioned flap with or without osseous surgery can be used to increase the clinical crown length.

A. If the tooth is periodontally healthy or affected by gingivitis only, crown lengthening can be accomplished by gingivectomy in cases of excess gingiva. This approach requires an adequate zone of attached gingiva with at least 3 mm of sound tooth structure above the crest of bone. If a mucogingival problem is anticipated, use an apically positioned flap to retain the available gingiva and lengthen the crown. A gingival graft is performed in instances of inadequate attached gingiva.

   Electrosurgery, an alternative to the gingivectomy, is a quick method for reducing excess tissue and providing good control of hemorrhage. Care must be taken to avoid contact with the bone. Even minimal contact with the alveolar process may result in overcoagulation, necrosis, resorption of bone, and gingival recession. In most circumstances use of a blade is preferable to an electrosurgical unit.

B. If the bone level is normal with no root fracture, use mucogingival-osseous surgery to expose at least 3 mm of root beyond where the restorative margin is to be placed. If a fracture extends into the root, assess the prognosis, accessibility, and esthetics before proceeding further. When a fracture compromises a furcation, root resection is a consideration. Extraction is indicated if the fracture extends to the middle third of the root or jeopardizes the support of the adjacent teeth. If the root fracture occurs in a more favorable location (coronal to the mid-third of the root), use a gingival flap with osseous surgery to expose the fractured area and create the appropriate biologic width.

   Maintenance of esthetics is a major concern in the anterior and premolar region. Orthodontics/forced eruption is a treatment option allowing extrusion of the fractured tooth with conservation of bone and esthetics; however, the need for periodontal surgery is not necessarily eliminated. Minimal crown lengthening to correct osseous contours then may be confined to the extruded tooth.

C. If the tooth requiring crown lengthening has periodontal pockets, assess the degree of periodontal support, strategic value, and prognosis using the same criteria outlined in B. Initial therapy is performed before crown lengthening to decrease inflammation and promote better hemostasis. Use mucogingival-osseous surgery to eliminate the periodontal pockets and to lengthen the crown.

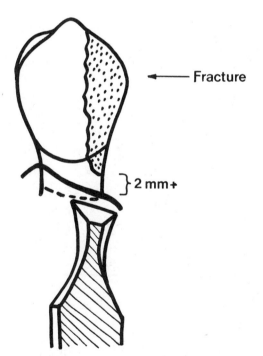

Fracture

2 mm+

Figure 1. When crown lengthening is performed where a fracture extends apically into the root, bone must be removed to expose a minimum of 2 mm of root structure apical to the ultimate margin of the restoration.

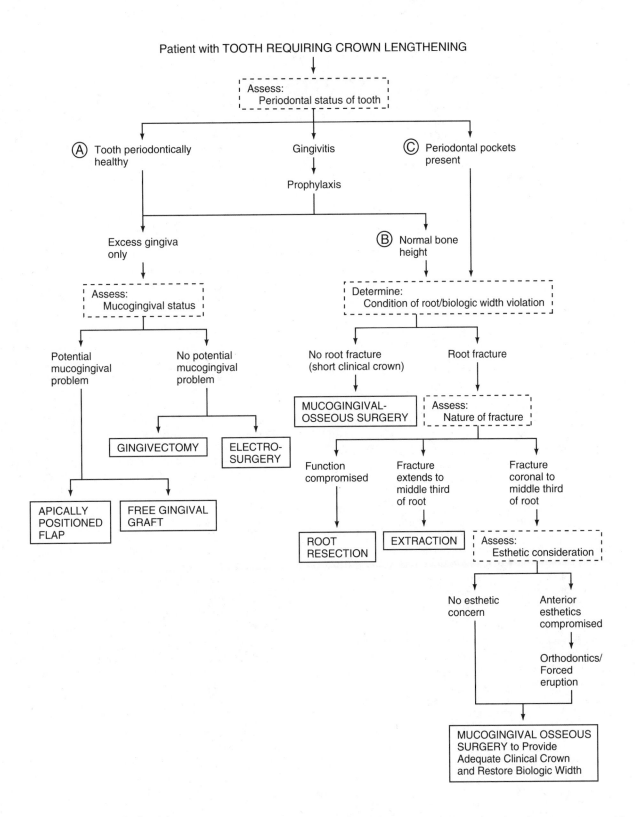

Patient with TOOTH REQUIRING CROWN LENGTHENING

Assess:
Periodontal status of tooth

Ⓐ Tooth periodontically healthy

Gingivitis

Ⓒ Periodontal pockets present

Prophylaxis

Excess gingiva only

Ⓑ Normal bone height

Assess:
Mucogingival status

Determine:
Condition of root/biologic width violation

Potential mucogingival problem

No potential mucogingival problem

No root fracture (short clinical crown)

Root fracture

GINGIVECTOMY

ELECTRO-SURGERY

MUCOGINGIVAL-OSSEOUS SURGERY

Assess:
Nature of fracture

APICALLY POSITIONED FLAP

FREE GINGIVAL GRAFT

Function compromised

Fracture extends to middle third of root

Fracture coronal to middle third of root

ROOT RESECTION

EXTRACTION

Assess:
Esthetic consideration

No esthetic concern

Anterior esthetics compromised

Orthodontics/ Forced eruption

MUCOGINGIVAL OSSEOUS SURGERY to Provide Adequate Clinical Crown and Restore Biologic Width

References

Johnson RH. Lengthening clinical crowns. J Am Dent Assoc 1990; 121(4):473.

Pruthi VK. Surgical crown lengthening in periodontics. J Can Dent Assoc 1987; 53(12):911.

Rosenberg M, Kay H, Keough B, Holt R. Periodontal and prosthetic management for advanced cases. Quintessence, 1988:164.

Sivers JE, Johnson GK. Periodontal and restorative considerations for crown lengthening. Quintessence Int 1985; 16(12):833.

Wagenberg B, Eskow R, Langer B. Exposing adequate tooth structure for restorative dentistry. Int J Periodontol Restor Dent, 1989; 9(5):323.

SELECTION OF THE APPROPRIATE PERIODONTAL SURGICAL TECHNIQUE

Walter B. Hall

When the dentist has determined that periodontal surgery is needed in the treatment of a complex dental case, he or the periodontist (to whom the patient may have been referred) must first determine the nature of the surgical problem. Periodontal surgical procedures may be regarded as pure mucogingival procedures or mucogingival-osseous procedures.

A. Pure mucogingival procedures include those whose goals are gingival augmentation when inadequate attached gingiva is present. These procedures (from most versatile to least) include the following: connective tissue graft, free gingival graft, and pedicle grafts. Ridge augmentation is a procedure used when no teeth are involved to create a better formed, more esthetic ridge on which to construct a bridge.

   The dentist must determine if recession is active in an area of inadequate gingiva, especially areas with less than 2 mm of attached gingiva. Earlier recordings, photographs, and old study models are more useful than the patient's impressions, though the latter may be all that is available. If recession can be documented as active, gingival augmentation is recommended. If not, the dentist must decide whether the proposed orthodontic or restorative treatment will require gingival augmentation. If so, he must discuss the advantages and disadvantages of augmentation with the patient and record his decisions. If the patient decides not to undergo gingival augmentation or if the orthodontic or restorative treatment does not indicate an immediate need for augmentation, the area may be maintained and a connective tissue graft for root coverage employed should recession occur.

B. Mucogingival-osseous problems are the result of inflammatory periodontal diseases that cause loss of attachment, bone loss, and pocket formation. These problems demand attention prior to restoration or orthodontics. Regaining lost attachment therefore is the most desirable goal.

C. Guided tissue regeneration has been demonstrated to be a predictable procedure in the presence of Class II furcas more than 3 mm horizontally between roots (but not through and through), three-walled osseous defects, or osseous craters (two-walled defects). Additional applications of the technique are expected to become predictable in the near future.

D. When lesions not predictably amenable to new attachment procedures are present, the dentist should consider the desirability of pocket elimination surgery prior to restoration or orthodontics (or in some cases [e.g., uprighting a tooth] after orthodontics). If the postsurgical results would be grotesque or unlikely to be more cleansible (or cleaned), a modified Widman flap, which does not result in pocket elimination, may be employed for thorough debridement and/or root modification prior to restoration. If the problem is relatively minimal and the patient demonstrably motivated, maintenance with frequent root planing alone may be the best option.

References

Carranza FA. Clinical periodontology. 7th ed. Philadelphia: WB Saunders, 1990:762.

Hall WB. Decision making in periodontology. 2nd ed. St Louis: Mosby, 1993:78.

Hall WB, Lundergan W. Free gingival grafts. Current indications and techniques. Dent Clin North Am 1993:227.

Schluger S, Yuodelis R, Page RC, Johnson RH. Periodontal diseases. 2nd ed. Philadelphia: Lea & Febiger, 1989:334.

Townsend, Olsen C, Ammons WF, van Bellen G. A longitudinal study comparing apically repositioned flaps with and without osseous surgery.

Patient with a COMPLEX DENTAL PROBLEM REQUIRING PERIODONTAL SURGERY

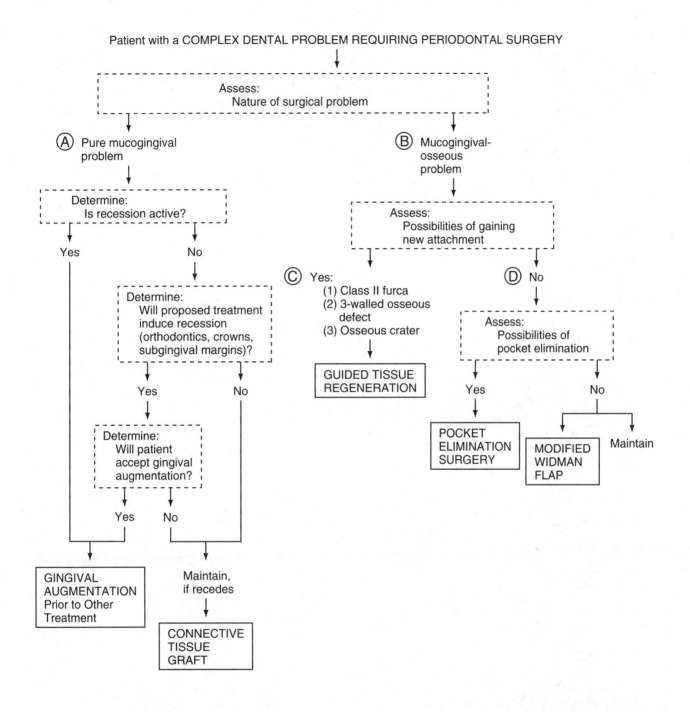

RIDGE PREPARATION

Walter B. Hall

When an edentulous area is present in the mouth of a patient with a complex dental problem, the treatment plan should include a means of restoring that area to function. The adequacy of the remaining edentulous ridge to support the proposed restoration becomes critically important early in the decision making process. As implants are always one option for restoring an edentulous area, a primary decision must be made as to the adequacy of the ridge to support implants either as replacement teeth or as abutments for a prosthesis. If the ridge is inadequate, the next decision involves whether it can be made adequate to support implants. If implants are not to be used, the adequacy of the ridge to support a selected prosthesis must be evaluated (Fig. 1, *A* to *C*).

A. If implants are to be employed, the adequacy of the ridge in terms of height and bulk of bone to support the implants must be evaluated. The presence of large maxillary sinuses beneath a thin plate of bone or the presence of a mandibular canal that would interfere with implant placement must be considered. If the ridge is adequate, implants may be placed individually or act as abutments for a prosthesis. Patient desire and cost are factors that may influence this decision as well.

B. If the ridge is not adequate for implant placement, some means of creating an adequate ridge may be employed. Guided tissue regeneration can regenerate bone to support implants on a predictable basis in many cases. It may be done in conjunction with the placement of the implants or, occasionally, before or afterward. In the presence of maxillary sinus with inadequate bone covering to permit implant placement, a sinus lift procedure may be used to increase the ridge bulk into which the implant is placed. A period of 6 months or so should be allowed before "permanent" restoration is undertaken. If neither of these approaches can be used, an alternative to implantation should be utilized.

C. If implants are not planned, the edentulous ridge should be evaluated to determine whether its existing form is adequate for restoration placement. Both form and esthetic aspects must be studied. If the ridge is adequate, restoration can proceed without surgical alteration.

D. If the ridge is misshapen or grotesque in form but adequate in bulk, ridgeplasty can be utilized to create a functionally and esthetically ideal or adequate form prior to restoration.

E. If the ridge is inadequate in bulk or form and would contribute to an unesthetic or poorly functional restoration, ridge augmentation is a newly predictable means of creating a more ideal ridge form prior to restoration.

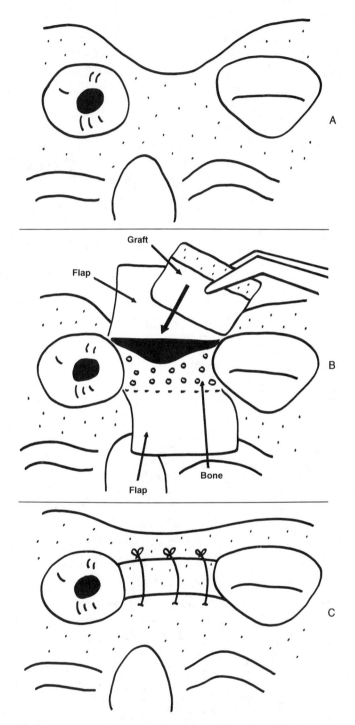

Figure 1. **A,** An incisal view of a disfigured ridge caused by loss of its facial cortical plate in an accident. **B,** Flaps have been raised, exposing the deficient ridge. A subepithelial connective tissue graft from the palate is being placed into the defect. **C,** The connective tissue graft has been sutured to fill the defect, plumping the ridge to create an esthetically pleasing base for a pontic.

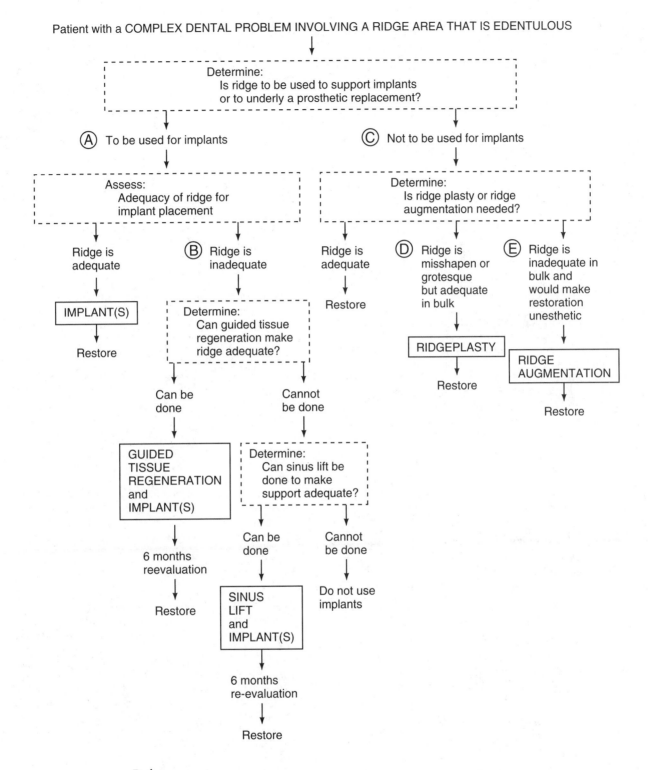

Patient with a COMPLEX DENTAL PROBLEM INVOLVING A RIDGE AREA THAT IS EDENTULOUS

Determine:
Is ridge to be used to support implants or to underly a prosthetic replacement?

(A) To be used for implants

Assess:
Adequacy of ridge for implant placement

Ridge is adequate

IMPLANT(S)

Restore

(B) Ridge is inadequate

Determine:
Can guided tissue regeneration make ridge adequate?

Can be done

Cannot be done

GUIDED TISSUE REGENERATION and IMPLANT(S)

6 months reevaluation

Restore

Determine:
Can sinus lift be done to make support adequate?

Can be done

Cannot be done

SINUS LIFT and IMPLANT(S)

6 months re-evaluation

Restore

Do not use implants

(C) Not to be used for implants

Determine:
Is ridge plasty or ridge augmentation needed?

Ridge is adequate

Restore

(D) Ridge is misshapen or grotesque but adequate in bulk

RIDGEPLASTY

Restore

(E) Ridge is inadequate in bulk and would make restoration unesthetic

RIDGE AUGMENTATION

Restore

References

Allen EP, Gainza CS, Farthing GC, Newbold DA. Improved technique for localized ridge augmentation: A report of 21 cases. J Periodontol 1985; 56:195.

Carranza FA. Clinical periodontology. 7th ed. Philadelphia: WB Saunders, 1990:922.

Hall WB. Periodontal preparation of the mouth for restoration. Dent Clin North Am 1980; 24:208.

Langer B, Calagna L. The subepithelial connective tissue graft. J Prosthet Dent 1980; 44:363.

Seibert J. Reconstruction of deformed, partially edentulous ridges using full thickness grafts: I—Technique and wound healing. Compend Contin Educ Dent 1983; 4:437.

Seibert J. Reconstruction of deformed, partially edentulous ridges using full thickness grafts. II. Prosthodontic/periodontal interrelationships. Compend Contin Educ Dent 1983; 4:549.

ESTABLISHING THE ADEQUACY OF ATTACHED GINGIVA

Walter B. Hall

When a tooth has a minimal amount of attached gingiva on either its facial or lingual surface, it is indicative of a potential pure mucogingival problem. The term "inadequate attached gingiva" was coined during the 1960s and has been defined loosely by many investigators. Rather than being a fixed number of millimeters of attached gingiva, it is a clinical estimate of the adequacy of the attached gingiva on an individual tooth to remain stable and healthy either under conditions imposed by any planned dental treatment or in the absence of any dental treatment involving the tooth (Fig. 1). The "attached gingiva" has been defined as ". . . that gingiva extending from the free margin of the gingiva to the mucogingival line minus the pocket or sulcus depth measured with a thin probe in the absence of inflammation" (Hall 1984). That the gingiva is "inadequate" in an individual case is a clinical decision made by the treating dentist based on a judgment of the tooth's needs within the patient's overall treatment plan. The decision on the need to treat is made with the concurrence of the informed patient (or parent).

A. A simple guideline for determining whether a pure mucogingival problem exists or not is to record all areas with less than 2 mm of total gingiva as potential problems because they have 1 mm or less attached gingiva when crevice depth is subtracted from the total gingiva. This does not mean that all such cases require grafting. Conversely, though a tooth may have more than 2 mm of total gingiva, it may still have 1 mm or less of attached gingiva when crevice depth is subtracted from total gingiva. In such a case its need for grafting would be determined as in any case with 1 mm or less of attached gingiva. It might require grafting if the tooth were to function as an abutment for a rest-proximal plate-I (RPI) bar-type removable partial denture or an overdenture.

B. For teeth with less than 1 mm of attached gingiva, the patient's age must be considered. Younger patients are more likely to require treatment than are older ones because of the longer period of time in which they would be expected to keep their teeth.

C. If a young patient has less than 1 mm of attached gingiva on a tooth and is having active recession (i.e., any root exposure at this age), consider grafting to stop further recession with a highly predictably successful graft on a periosteal bed rather than awaiting the necessity to perform a graft at a later time whose success would depend on new attachment to an exposed root. If the young patient has no recession but a restorative procedure (such as Class V restoration) or orthodontic treatment is planned, consider grafting prophylactically. If no such restorative or orthodontic work is planned, observe the area for change at all future visits rather than grafting at this time. If the patient is older and has less than 1 mm of attached gingiva on a tooth and active recession, consider grafting at this time. If the situation appears stable (with or without root exposure), the need to treat depends on restorative or orthodontic plans. If crowns, bridges, RPI partials, or overdentures involving this tooth are planned or if orthodontic work is planned, consider grafting; if not, observe the area for evidence of change.

D. If the patient has 2 mm or more of attached gingiva on a tooth that cannot serve as an abutment for an RPI removable partial or an overdenture, grafting need not be considered. If such a restoration is planned, however, the tooth may require grafting either to create at least 3 mm of attached gingiva over which the RPI clasp would be positioned or to support the movement resulting from an overdenture. If the tooth has 3 mm or more of attached gingiva, grafting is unlikely to be needed.

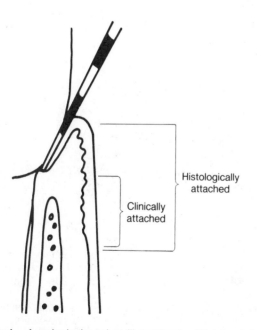

Figure 1. A probe in the sulcus illustrating the difference between clinically and histologically attached gingiva.

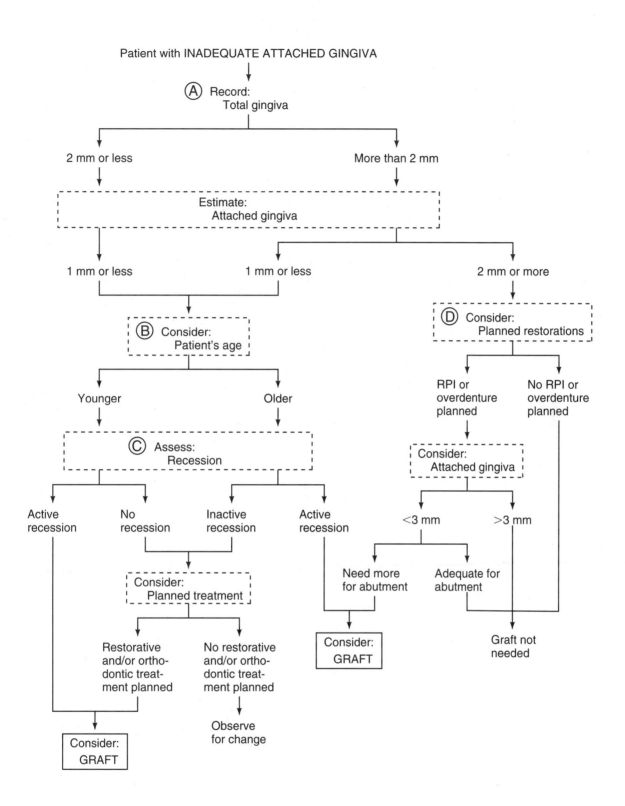

Patient with INADEQUATE ATTACHED GINGIVA

Ⓐ Record:
Total gingiva

2 mm or less   More than 2 mm

Estimate:
Attached gingiva

1 mm or less   1 mm or less   2 mm or more

Ⓑ Consider:
Patient's age

Ⓓ Consider:
Planned restorations

Younger   Older

RPI or overdenture planned   No RPI or overdenture planned

Ⓒ Assess:
Recession

Consider:
Attached gingiva

Active recession   No recession   Inactive recession   Active recession

<3 mm   >3 mm

Consider:
Planned treatment

Need more for abutment   Adequate for abutment

Restorative and/or orthodontic treatment planned   No restorative and/or orthodontic treatment planned

Consider:
GRAFT

Graft not needed

Observe for change

Consider:
GRAFT

References

Hall WB. Present status of soft tissue grafting. J Periodontol 1977; 48:587.

Hall WB. Pure mucogingival problems. Berlin: Quintessence Publishing, 1984:61.

Lang NP, Loe H. The relationship between the width of the attached gingiva and gingival health. J Periodontol 1972; 43:623.

Lindhe J. Textbook of clinical periodontology. 2nd ed. Copenhagen: Munksgaard, 1989:422.

Maynard JG, Wilson RDK. Physiologic dimensions of the periodontium significant to the restorative dentist. J Periodontol 1979; 50:170.

World Workshop in Clinical Periodontics. Chicago: American Academy of Periodontology, 1989:VII-10, VII-16, VII-17.

GINGIVAL AUGMENTATION

Giovan Paolo Pini-Prato
Carlo Clauser
Pierpaolo Cortellini

A. Restoration margins in periodontally involved patients should be supragingival whenever possible. The subgingival placement of margins may be indicated for cosmetic reasons, but it induces inflammation and compromises the ability to control plaque (Hall 1989).

B. Plaque accumulation induces an inflammatory response with infiltrate in the supracrestal connective tissue. This response is not related to the width of the gingiva (Lindhe 1983). On the other hand, the thickness of the gingiva is critical for recession and visual signs of inflammation. A thick free gingiva is less prone to recession than a thin one in the presence of subgingival plaque (Erickson and Lindhe 1984) and may hide both the prosthetic margin and the intracrevicular inflammatory reaction. Because both recession and reddening of the gingival margin are detrimental to the cosmetic appearance, they must be avoided when cosmetic considerations have indicated subgingival placement of the restorative margin. In other words, the subgingival placement of a restoration margin requires a rather thick free gingiva.

C. The thickness of the gingiva is difficult to assess directly, but it is related to its width. A keratinized tissue width of at least 2 mm has been reported to be associated with lower gingival scores in the presence of subgingival restoration margins (Stetler and Bissada 1987).

D. The term *gingiva* usually refers to the keratinized tissue surrounding natural teeth. Because the role and the relationships of peri-implant and edentulous ridge tissues are different, the term *keratinized tissue* may be preferable when dealing with edentulous areas.

E. The need for attached keratinized tissue around osteointegrated implants is controversial (Adell et al. 1981; Schroeder et al. 1981). Even if an implant can be maintained in spite of the presence of movable alveolar mucosa around its neck, the most desirable situation seems to be a region of immobile keratinized mucosa around the implant, especially where monophasic plasma-sprayed implants are concerned.

Patient with a COMPLEX DENTAL PROBLEM AND INADEQUATE GINGIVA IN SOME AREAS

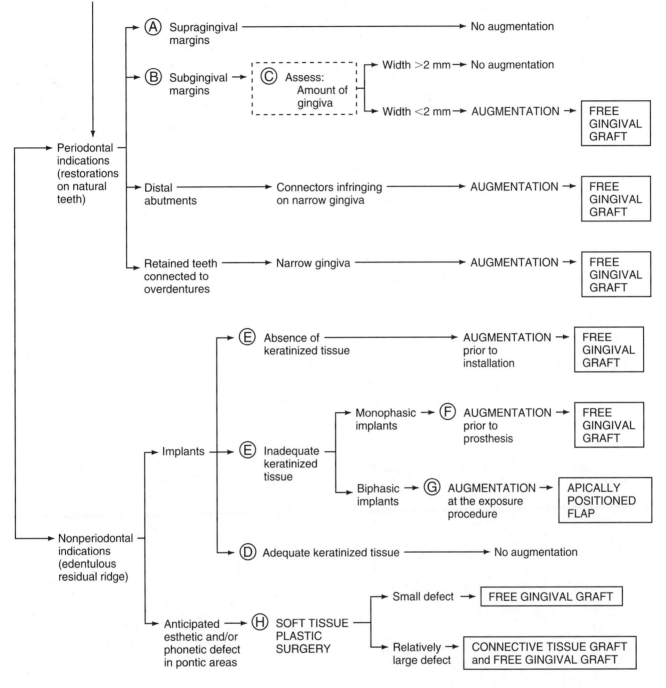

F. Free gingival grafts are indicated if a monophasic (not submerged) implant has an inadequate amount of keratinized tissue, preferably prior to the connection with the final prosthetic reconstruction. In cases of extreme reduction of the keratinized tissue the grafting procedure should be carried out prior to implant installation (Buser 1991).

G. If a submerged implant has been installed in an area of narrow keratinized tissue, an augmentation procedure is indicated, preferably at the same time as the surgical exposure of the implant body. An apically positioned flap allows keratinized tissue augmentation while exposing the implants, thus saving all the available tissue (Fig. 1).

H. Soft tissue plastic surgery (Pini-Prato and De Sanctis 1991) is indicated to restore an acceptable profile in localized edentulous areas that need to be restored by conventional crown and bridge restorations, provided that the ridge does not have to withstand masticatory load. Two stage procedures including connective tissue grafts may correct horizontal and/or vertical defects. Free gingival grafts are indicated in cases of small defects (Fig. 2). Major preprosthetic surgery or hard tissue reconstruction is indicated to treat alveolar ridge deficiencies. See Fig. 3, *A* to *D*.

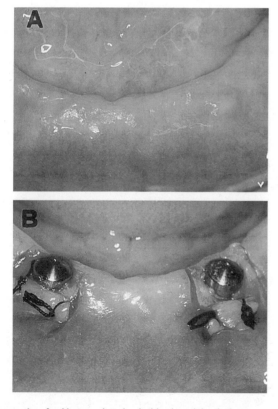

Figure 1. **A,** Narrow band of thin keratinized tissue on the edentulous ridge over two submerged implants. **B,** The implants are exposed via apically positioned flap.

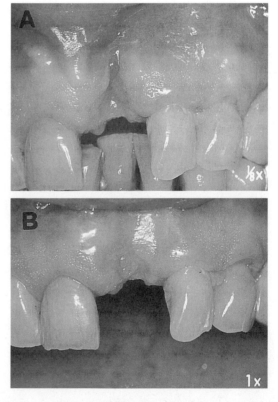

Figure 2. **A,** Ridge deficiency after extraction of a periodontally involved maxillary central incisor. **B,** The same site after free gingival graft.

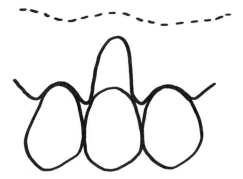

Figure 3. A, A localized recession requiring gingival augmentation for root coverage.

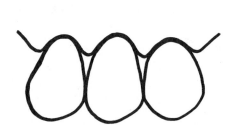

Figure 3. D, The healed area with full root coverage.

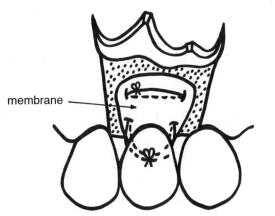

membrane

Figure 3. B, A GoreTex membrane with supporting strut suture covering the prepared receptor site.

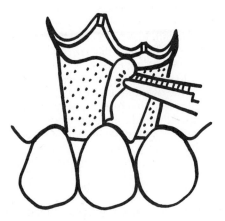

Figure 3. C, Removal of the GoreTex membrane to reveal regeneration tissue covering the root.

References

Adell B, Lekholm U, Rockler B, Branemark PI. A 15 year study of osteointegrated implants in the treatment of edentulous jaw. Int J Oral Surg 1981; 10:387.

Buser D. Mucogingival surgery. In: Schroeder A, Sutter F, Krekeler G, eds. Oral implantology. Basics—III. Hollow cylinder system. Stuttgart: Georg Thieme Verlag; 1991:295.

Erickson I, Lindhe J. Recession in sites with inadequate width of keratinized gingiva. An experimental study in the dog. J Clin Periodontol 1984; 11:95.

Hall WB. Gingival augmentation/mucogingival surgery. In: World Workshop in Clinical Periodontics. Chicago: American Academy of Periodontology, 1989:VII-1.

Lindhe J: Textbook of clinical periodontology. Copenhagen: Munksgaard, 1983.

Pini Prato GP, De Sanctis M. Soft tissue plastic surgery. Current Opin Dent 1991; 1:98.

Schroeder A, van der Zypen E, Stich H. The reactions of bone, connective tissue and epithelium to endosteal implants with titanium sprayed surfaces. J Oral Maxillofac Surg 1981; 9:15.

Stetler KJ, Bissada NF. Significance of the width of keratinized gingiva on the periodontal status of teeth with submarginal restorations. J Periodontol 1987; 58:696.

RESTORATIVE PLANS AND GINGIVAL GRAFTING

Walter B. Hall

When a tooth that is predisposed to recession by lack of adequate attached gingiva has restorative needs or is to be used as an abutment, the dentist must decide whether grafting to increase the band of attached gingiva is indicated or not. If the patient elects not to proceed with a graft when indicated, he must be informed of the potential problems.

A. If the predisposed tooth requires restoration, the type of restoration and its locale are most important. If a class V restoration is to be supragingival, there is no need to graft. If the class V restoration is to be close to the gingival margin or subgingival, a graft should be considered. If the restoration is to be of any other class, grafting need not be considered.

B. If the predisposed tooth requires a crown and the crown margins are to be supragingival, there is no need to graft; however, if the crown margin is to be placed at the gingival margin or subgingivally, grafting is indicated because the diamond bur will cut soft tissue as well as tooth structure when carried subgingivally and will produce recession as a consequence of the soft tissue curettage. If the entire crown of the tooth is to be visible and recession would expose a chamfer, the patient must be made aware that not grafting is likely to result in a visible gold margin apical to the porcelain facing. Grafting beforehand should be strongly encouraged, because covering an exposed chamfer surgically after crown placement is exceedingly unlikely to be successful.

C. If the predisposed tooth is to become an abutment for a fixed bridge, grafting should be considered whether or not a subgingival margin is to be placed in the area of inadequate attached gingiva. Cleaning under the pontic or between it and the tooth is likely to produce recession. If a three-quarter crown design is to be employed, grafting should be considered but is not as essential as when a full crown restoration is to be placed.

D. If the predisposed tooth is to serve as an abutment for a rest-proximal plate-I (RPI) bar-type removable partial denture, a sufficiently large enough graft should be placed such that the entire I-bar will be over the gingiva. If this is not done, the patient who removes the partial denture by placing a fingernail under the apical end of the I-bar is likely to cause wounding and to induce recession (Fig. 1). A graft usually cannot be placed under an existing I-bar, because the space is inadequate for a graft of sufficient thickness to be placed; therefore a new partial denture needs to be constructed following grafting.

E. If the predisposed tooth is to be used as an abutment for an overdenture, much the same situation applies. If recession occurs (which is likely when a full denture is placed in the area), the denture could be relieved and a graft placed or the denture could be left out while the graft heals. In either case the graft is likely to be moved about and to fail. Instead, a large flange of acrylic must be cut away, the graft placed, and the overdenture rebased once healing is completed. A more advisable course is to graft on any predisposed tooth prior to beginning the overdenture treatment. If a graft is to be placed for restorative reasons, selection of the type to be employed would involve consideration of the options among free gingival grafts, pedicle grafts, or connective tissue grafts (see p 50).

References

Genco EJ, Goldman HM, Cohen DW. Contemporary periodontics. St Louis: CV Mosby, 1990:621.

Hall WB. Periodontal preparation of the mouth for restoration. Dent Clin North Am 1980; 24:195.

Hall WB. Pure mucogingival problems. Berlin: Quintessence Publishing, 1984:41.

Maynard JG, Wilson RD: Physiologic dimensions of the periodontium significant to the restorative dentist. J Periodontol 1979; 50:170.

World Workshop in Clinical Periodontics. Chicago: American Academy of Periodontology, 1989:VII-16.

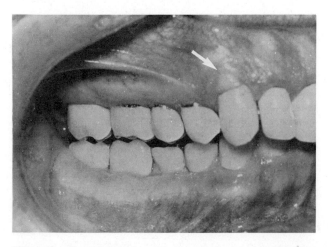

Figure 1. Recession of 3 mm has occurred on the canine (which had inadequate attached gingiva) following crown placement.

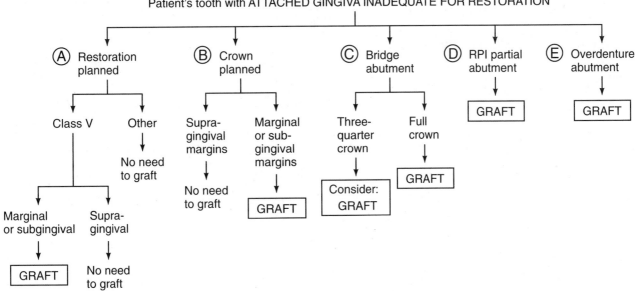

Patient's tooth with ATTACHED GINGIVA INADEQUATE FOR RESTORATION

Ⓐ Restoration planned

Class V

Marginal or subgingival

GRAFT

Supra-gingival

No need to graft

Other

No need to graft

Ⓑ Crown planned

Supra-gingival margins

No need to graft

Marginal or sub-gingival margins

GRAFT

Ⓒ Bridge abutment

Three-quarter crown

Consider: GRAFT

Full crown

GRAFT

Ⓓ RPI partial abutment

GRAFT

Ⓔ Overdenture abutment

GRAFT

RECESSION TREATMENT: ROOT COVERAGE OR NOT?

Walter B. Hall

When a patient has a root or roots exposed by recession, esthetic and restorative considerations influence the need for grafting in an interrelated manner. If the band of attached gingiva is adequate but recession has occurred, surgery may be utilized to recover exposed roots for esthetic reasons. If no esthetic need exists and no restoration affecting the gingival margin is planned, maintenance care alone should suffice. If the band of attached gingiva is inadequate in the dentist's opinion, the need to consider gingival augmentation is greater (Figs. 1 to 5).

A. First decide upon the "adequacy" of the existing band of attached gingiva. An adequate band of attached gingiva is sufficient to prevent initial or continued recession. The patient's age, other dental needs, oral hygiene status, caries activity, and esthetic needs are factors that influence a decision that treatment is needed to prevent initial or continued recession if the band of attached gingiva is judged to be inadequate.

B. If the patient has an adequate band of attached gingiva and no cosmetic or esthetic need to attempt root coverage exists, dental health should be maintainable with regular oral hygiene, prophylaxis, and/or root planing. If a class V restoration or crown is to be placed, the apical margin of the restoration may be placed within the gingival crevice without strong likelihood of inducing recession or it may be placed supragingivally. If root sensitivity, caries activity, or other restorative requirements (e.g., crown length) are not involved, then maintenance care should suffice.

C. If root coverage is necessary to meet esthetic or cosmetic goals, and if the band of attached gingiva on the tooth or teeth with recession is adequate, a coronally positioned pedicle graft or flap (see p 50) is the treatment of choice.

D. When an inadequate band of attached gingiva is present and esthetic cosmetic or restorative goals indicate the need for root coverage, a coronally positioned pedicle graft (flap) is not likely to be successful. In this situation a connective tissue graft is most appropriate, particularly if several teeth are involved. If an adequate donor site for such a graft is not available (i.e., the donor site in the rugae area is insufficiently thick), then pedicle grafts should be considered.

E. If the patient has inadequate attached gingiva to meet his dental needs without initiating recession or further recession and no cosmetic or esthetic concern exists, a free gingival graft without root coverage may be performed for stabilization.

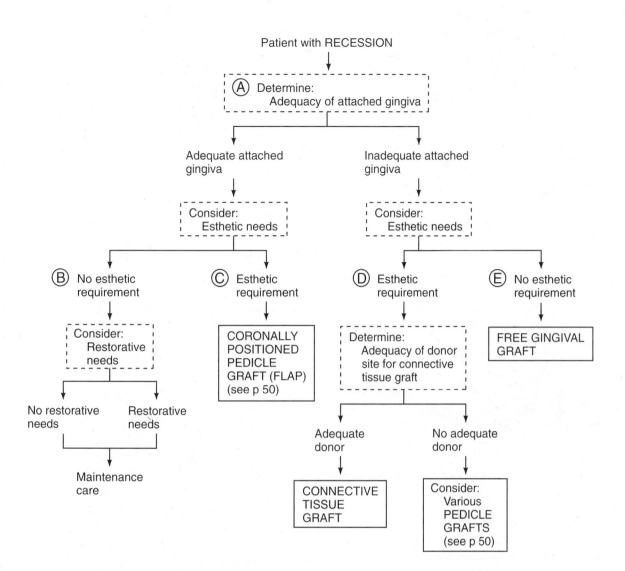

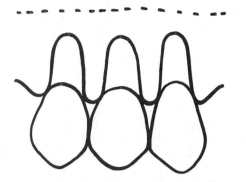

Figure 1. Multiple adjacent teeth with gingival recession to be treated with a subepithelial connective tissue (CT) graft.

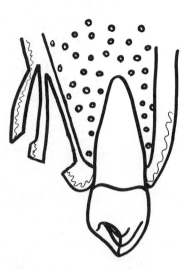

Figure 3. Sagittal view of the palatal donor area showing the primary and secondary (CT graft) flaps prepared.

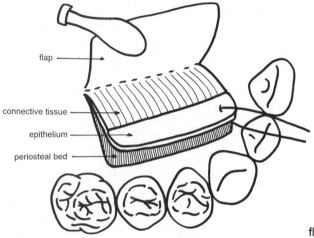

flap

connective tissue

epithelium

periosteal bed

Figure 2. Obtaining the CT graft from the palate.

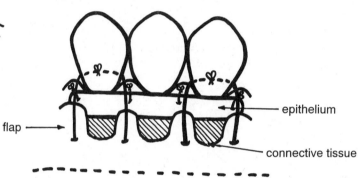

epithelium

flap

connective tissue

Figure 4. The CT graft sutured to cover the exposed roots with the receptor site flap positioned covering much of the connective tissue.

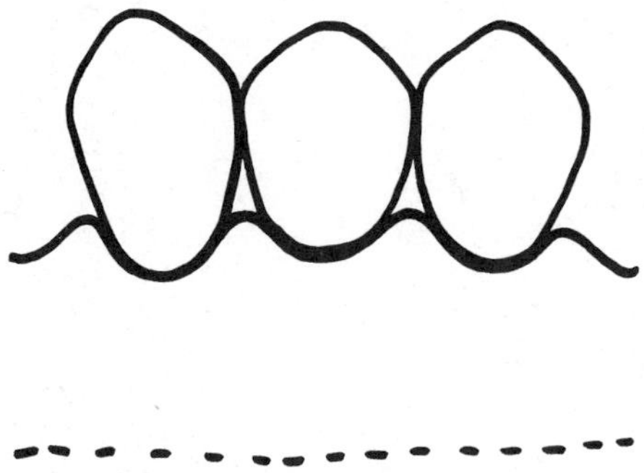

Figure 5. The healed area with full root coverage.

References

Allen EP, Miller PD. Coronal positioning of existing gingiva: Short term results in the treatment of shallow marginal tissue recession. J Periodontol 1989; 60:316.

Langer B, Langer L. Subepithelial connective tissue graft technique for root coverage. J Periodontol 1985; 56:715.

Hall WB. Pure mucogingival problems. Berlin: Quintessence Publishing, 1984:61, 153.

Matter J. Free gingival grafts for the treatment of gingival recession—A review of some techniques. J Clin Periodontol 1980; 9:103.

World Workshop in Clinical Periodontics. Chicago: American Academy of Periodontology, 1989:VII-1, VII-17.

SELECTION OF GINGIVAL AUGMENTATION TECHNIQUES

Walter B. Hall

Once a decision has been made that a pure mucogingival problem requires surgery to create a broader band of attached gingiva, the dentist must select the technique most likely to achieve root coverage or a broader band of attached gingiva to minimize recession in the future. Esthetics is a prime consideration. Connective tissue grafts and pedicle grafts are more likely than free grafts to be successful in covering roots and in matching the appearance of adjacent gingiva. Connective tissue grafting appears to be more successful than pedicle grafting; therefore, when root coverage is a goal, the connective tissue graft would be preferable to any pedicle graft procedure unless an adequately thick donor site for a connective tissue graft is not available (see p 46). See Figs. 1 and 2.

A. If no esthetic concern exists, as in most mandibular areas and in maxillary molar areas, a free gingival graft is one option. When no recession requiring coverage is present, a free gingival graft is an acceptable choice.

B. When no esthetic problem exists but recession requiring root coverage is present or when an esthetic problem is present, a connective tissue graft or a pedicle graft should be utilized for root coverage and for a better esthetic result. Connective tissue grafts have a higher degree of predictability of success than do pedicle grafts; uninvolved is going to be extracted (i.e., some first premolars), no augmentation procedure for that area is indicated.

If no orthodontic treatment is planned, restorative needs also may influence the need for gingival augmentation. If no Class V restoration or crown is planned in the predisposed area, its current status should be documented; if recession occurs, a connective tissue graft (or, alternatively, a pedicle graft) is employed to stop further recession and cover some or all of the exposed root. If a Class V restoration or crown is indicated on a predisposed tooth where less than 1 mm of recession has occurred, the patient may elect a free gingival graft to augment the inadequate band of attached gingiva; alternatively, the patient may take his chances; if recession does occur, the less predictable connective tissue graft (or pedicle graft) can be placed to stop further recession and cover the newly exposed root in whole or in part.

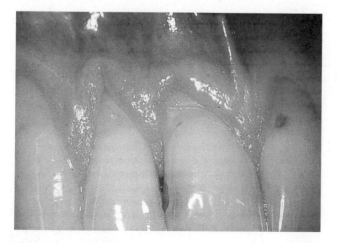

Figure 1. Preoperative view of an area with recession on several teeth where root coverage is indicated.

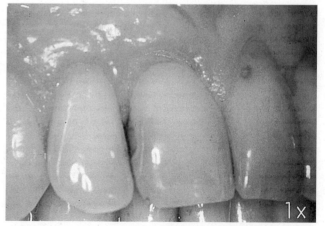

Figure 2. Postoperative view of successful gingival augmentation 1 year later.

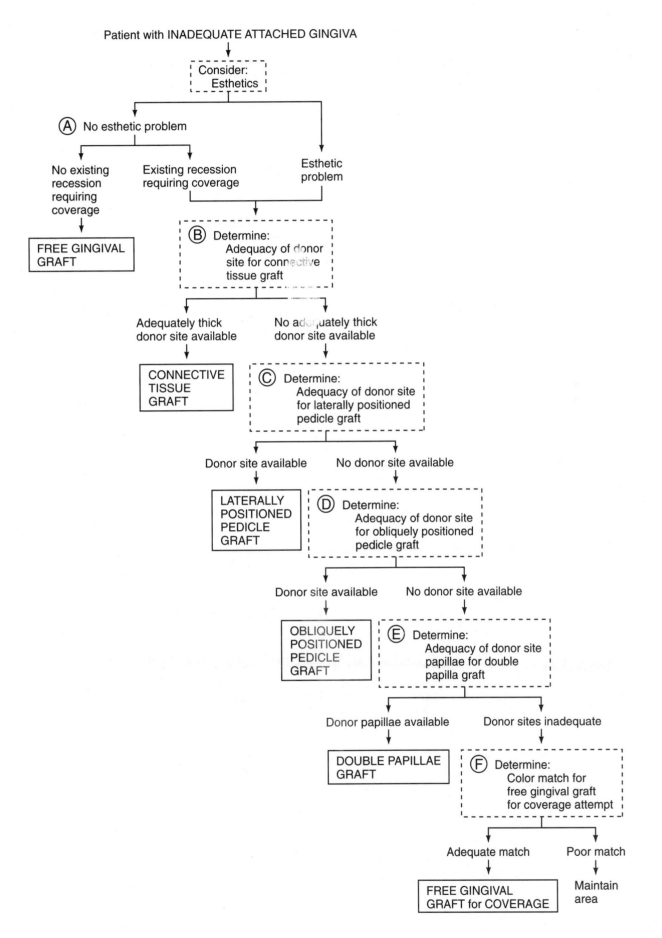

Patient with INADEQUATE ATTACHED GINGIVA

Consider:
Esthetics

(A) No esthetic problem

No existing recession requiring coverage

Existing recession requiring coverage

Esthetic problem

FREE GINGIVAL GRAFT

(B) Determine:
Adequacy of donor site for connective tissue graft

Adequately thick donor site available

No adequately thick donor site available

CONNECTIVE TISSUE GRAFT

(C) Determine:
Adequacy of donor site for laterally positioned pedicle graft

Donor site available

No donor site available

LATERALLY POSITIONED PEDICLE GRAFT

(D) Determine:
Adequacy of donor site for obliquely positioned pedicle graft

Donor site available

No donor site available

OBLIQUELY POSITIONED PEDICLE GRAFT

(E) Determine:
Adequacy of donor site papillae for double papilla graft

Donor papillae available

Donor sites inadequate

DOUBLE PAPILLAE GRAFT

(F) Determine:
Color match for free gingival graft for coverage attempt

Adequate match

Poor match

FREE GINGIVAL GRAFT for COVERAGE

Maintain area

C. The laterally positioned graft has the highest likelihood of success. To use it, a donor site on adjacent teeth must be sufficiently wide, tall, and thick to be able to be raised as a flap of approximately 0.5 to 1.0 mm in thickness and laterally positioned to cover the exposed root (or potentially exposed area) with several millimeters of soft tissue on either side of it. The donor site should be about 1.5 times the width of the area to be covered and 2 to 5 mm in height. If such a donor site is not available, consider the next alternative.

D. An obliquely rotated pedicle graft can be used occasionally when an adequate donor site for a laterally positioned pedicle graft is not present. A papilla adjacent to the receptor area may be of sufficient width and height to be used as a donor site. The pedicle graft will be rotated about 90 degrees to cover the exposed (or potentially exposed) area; therefore the papilla should be tall enough to cover the receptor site plus at least a millimeter more mesiodistally. It also should be wide enough to provide sufficient gingiva to cover the exposed root or to achieve an adequate band of gingiva to minimize

recession in the future. The papilla may be taken full thickness, if necessary, as it overlies interproximal bone, which has a cancellous component subjacent to the cortical plate. It should not have a deep gingival groove, however, or it may split in two when raised. If no adequate donor site for such a graft exists, consider the next alternative.

E. A double papilla graft is the most difficult of the pedicle grafts to do and is the most likely to fail. The patient should understand these problems before proceeding (see p 6). The donor sites for such a graft are the two adjacent papillae. These papillae must be sufficiently wide when joined to cover the receptor site and extend a millimeter or more on each of the adjacent papillary donor sites. They should be tall enough to provide a sufficient band of attached gingiva to cover the exposed root or to minimize recession. As with obliquely positioned pedicle grafts, thickness is not a problem, but deep gingival grooves can make this approach untenable. When the donor sites are not sufficient, a free gingival graft should be considered.

F. Free gingival grafts for covering roots have long been a desired goal of those practicing pure mucogingival surgery; however, the predictability of success with a free graft is not great although claims for improved success with root treatment either with citric acid or complicated suturing have been made. The free gingival graft usually is taken from the palate, which may be of a markedly different color than the gingiva adjacent to the area to be grafted. If the donor gingiva is of such poor color match that it would create a greater esthetic problem than that created by root exposure, grafting for root coverage should not be attempted.

References

Carranza FA. Clinical periodontology. 7th ed., Philadelphia: WB Saunders, 1990:883, 893.

Hall WB. Pure mucogingival problems. Berlin: Quintessence Publishing, 1984:129.

Langer B, Langer L. Subepithelial connective tissue graft technique for root coverage. J Periodontol 1983; 56:175.

World Workshop in Clinical Periodontics. Chicago: American Academy of Periodontology, 1989:VII-1.

SELECTION OF MUCOGINGIVAL-OSSEOUS SURGICAL APPROACHES: RESECTION OR REGENERATION

Walter B. Hall

Many patients with complex dental problems require mucogingival-osseous surgery. Most have been affected by adult periodontitis and have a number of teeth with pocket depth, bone loss, and loss of attachment. The character of the bone loss present determines the type of mucogingival-osseous surgery indicated.

A. The dentist must first decide whether the problem is one of horizontal bone loss only, vertical loss only, or a mixed problem (some teeth with horizontal and some with vertical bone loss). If the patient has only horizontal bone loss, the severity of loss and the number of severely involved teeth are the factors that determine the treatment plan. If many teeth are severely affected, mucogingival-osseous surgery is contraindicated. The teeth should either be extracted or given a hopeless prognosis and maintained. The restorative plan is determined by which if any teeth could be utilized. If the horizontal bone loss is not severe or generalized, pocket elimination surgery with osteoplasty to create the most readily maintainable contours is best.

B. If vertical bone loss is involved, the types of osseous defects present determine the type of surgery indicated. One-walled defects that are shallow should be managed with pocket elimination surgery and osseous resection (osteoctomy and osteoplasty). If a one-walled defect is moderate to deep, the value of the individual tooth to the overall treatment plan should be considered. If the tooth is of little value, extraction

is the best approach. If the tooth is critical to the overall treatment plan, guided tissue regeneration with or without concomitant or second-stage osseous resection should be employed.

C. For two-walled defects the surgical approach depends on whether the defects are craters (defects between adjacent teeth where facial and lingual cortical plates remain) or the less common type affecting only one tooth (either a facial or a lingual cortical plate and a wall against the adjacent tooth remain). If a crater is present and is a shallow defect, pocket elimination surgery with osseous resection is best. If the crater is moderate to deep, guided tissue regeneration should be employed. If the two-walled defect affects only a single tooth, its value to the overall treatment plan determines whether guided tissue regeneration or extraction is best. See Figs. 1 and 2.

D. For three-walled defects the depth and horizontal width from root to osseous crest are the factors that determine the surgical approach. A narrow defect (less than 1 mm horizontally from root to osseous crest) is amenable to a "Prichard fill" technique wherein total debridement is followed by bone fill and new attachment on a predictable basis. If the defect is wide (more than 1 mm horizontally from root to osseous crest) and moderate to deep, guided tissue regeneration is a predicable means of gaining new attachment. If the defect is wide and shallow, pocket elimination with osseous resection is best.

BEFORE

AFTER

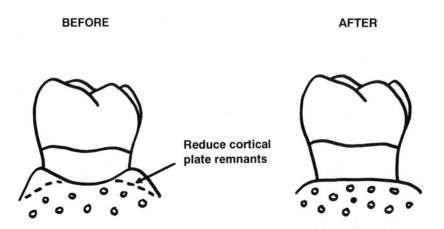

Reduce cortical plate remnants

Figure 1. A shallow two-walled infrabony "crater" is treated by osseous resection.

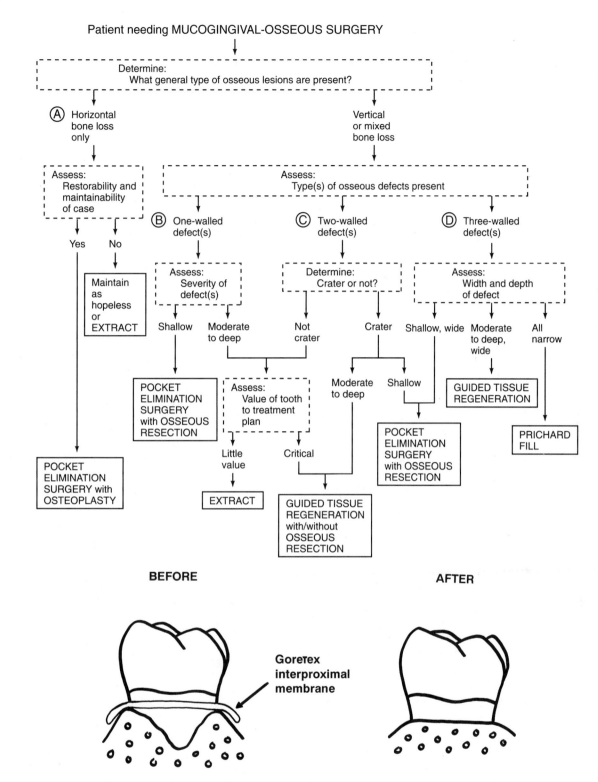

Patient needing MUCOGINGIVAL-OSSEOUS SURGERY

Determine:
What general type of osseous lesions are present?

Ⓐ Horizontal bone loss only

Vertical or mixed bone loss

Assess:
Restorability and maintainability of case

Assess:
Type(s) of osseous defects present

Yes   No

Ⓑ One-walled defect(s)

Ⓒ Two-walled defect(s)

Ⓓ Three-walled defect(s)

Maintain as hopeless or EXTRACT

Assess:
Severity of defect(s)

Determine:
Crater or not?

Assess:
Width and depth of defect

Shallow   Moderate to deep

Not crater   Crater

Shallow, wide   Moderate to deep, wide   All narrow

POCKET ELIMINATION SURGERY with OSSEOUS RESECTION

Assess:
Value of tooth to treatment plan

Moderate to deep   Shallow

GUIDED TISSUE REGENERATION

PRICHARD FILL

Little value   Critical

POCKET ELIMINATION SURGERY with OSSEOUS RESECTION

POCKET ELIMINATION SURGERY with OSTEOPLASTY

EXTRACT

GUIDED TISSUE REGENERATION with/without OSSEOUS RESECTION

BEFORE

AFTER

Goreᴛex interproximal membrane

Figure 2.   A deep two-walled infrabony "crater" is treated by guided tissue regeneration.

References

Carranza FA. Clinical periodontology. 7th ed. Philadelphia: WB Saunders, 1990:792.

Genco RJ, Goldman HM, Cohen DW. Contemporary periodontics. St Louis: CV Mosby, 1990:564, 585.

Knowles JW. Results of periodontal treatment related to pocket depth and attachment level: Eight years. J Periodontol 1979; 50:225.

Pihlstrom BJ, McHugh RB, Oliphant TH, Ortiz-Campos C. Comparison of surgical and non-surgical treatment of periodontal disease. J Clin Periodontol 1983; 10:524.

Schluger S, Yuodelis R, Page RC, Johnson RH. Periodontal diseases. 2nd ed. Philadelphia: Lea & Febiger, 1989:332.

Smith DH, Ammons WF, Van Belle G. A longitudinal study of periodontal status comparing osseous recontouring with flap curettage: 1—Results after 6 months. J Periodontol 1980; 51:367.

GUIDED TISSUE REGENERATION VERSUS OSSEOUS FILL

Mark D. Sutter

Once the decision to regenerate an area has been reached, the next decisions relate to how the osseous morphology, existing anatomy, patient selection, and future restorative concerns affect which procedure or combination is utilized.

A. Bone fill in infrabony defects with an infrabony technique and flap debridement can only occur if the defect is a narrow (1 mm from root to bone crest horizontally), three-walled vertical defect. As the width and absence of osseous walls contained within the osseous defect increases, bone fill becomes less predictable; therefore, the utilization of bone grafting and/or guided tissue regeneration to enhance regeneration should be considered. The osseous morphology of the periodontal defect is essential in determining the prospect for regeneration. Attachment loss of at least 4 mm should be present. As the depth, number, and narrowness of the infrabony walls increases, the potential for successful regeneration is more favorable. One-walled defects provide the least surface area.

   When evaluating the possibility of regeneration in teeth involved with furcations, the buccal, lingual and interproximal crestal bone should be of sufficient height to retain the gingival tissues as far above the roof of the furcation as possible. The closer the interproximal bone height is to the roof of the furcation, the poorer the potential for furcal resolution. *Class III furcation defects are the outer limit of predictable treatment.* Shallow osseous defects and class III (through and through) furcas should be treated by alternative means.

B. When extensive restorations, decay, or root perforations or fractures exist within the proposed area of regeneration, an alternative periodontal procedure may be necessary. When osseous resection does not compromise reasonable support, it may be the treatment of choice.

C. Certain medical conditions (e.g., valvular heart disease, prosthetic joint replacement, poorly controlled diabetes, heart murmurs, or a compromised immune system) may increase the risk of complications with the use of membrane techniques. Bone grafting or other conventional periodontal therapy should be evaluated in these cases.

D. Maxillary and mandibular anteriors often have thin gingival tissues that may be prone to recession and esthetic compromise. Alteration in blood supply leading to flap necrosis can occur, especially with guided tissue regeneration. Root proximity in maxillary molar and lower incisor areas may inhibit access for debridement and limit graft and/or membrane placement, as may fused roots, short root trunks, or unfavorable grooves and fissures.

Mandibular tori and thick cortical ledges favor regeneration. Their removal provides a ready source of autogenous bone and may allow the coronal repositioning of tissues for membrane coverage. Soft tissue coverage in any regenerative procedure is favorable, especially where bone grafting is to be utilized, because it facilitates containment of the bone grafting material within the defect. Defects adjacent to edentulous areas are excellent recipient sites for regenerative therapy as tissue coverage is maximized. Narrow interproximal sites often lack sufficient tissue for graft containment or barrier coverage.

E. Membrane techniques combined with bone grafting material favors regeneration by retarding epithelial downgrowth and by permitting osteogenesis to occur by the incorporation of an inductive bone grafting material. Utilizing both barrier and grafting technologies enhances predictability by facilitating graft containment and preventing membrane collapse, especially in treating infrabony, furcation, ridge, and even crestal and dehiscence defects.

   Two categories of osseous implant materials are available today. Regeneration-enhancing materials offer the possibility of regaining lost cementum, periodontal ligament, and bone. They include autogenous cancellous and cortical bone from either an oral or extraoral source and freeze-dried or demineralized freeze-dried bone allografts. In the other category, alloplasts offer only "filler potential" when used in periodontal defects. No evidence of a new attachment apparatus has been found with alloplasts. Examples of alloplastic materials include hydroxyapatite and tricalcium phosphate ceramics.

F. Guided tissue regeneration without osteogenic materials is discussed elsewhere (see p 62).

References

Anderegg CR. Clinical evaluation of the use of decalcified freeze-dried bone allograft with GTR in the treatment of molar furcation invasions. J Periodontol 1991; 62:264.

Bowers G. Histologic evaluation of new attachment apparatus formation in humans. Parts I, II and III. J Periodontol 1989; 60:664.

Ellegaard B. New attachment of periodontal tissues after treatment of infrabony lesions. J Periodontol 1971; 42:648.

Pontoriero R. Guided tissue regeneration in degree II furcation involved mandibular molars. A clinical study. J Clin Periodontol 1988; 15:247.

Pritchard JF. The infrabony technique as a predictable procedure. J Periodontol 1952; 28:202.

Schallhorn R. Combined osseous composite grafting, root conditioning and guided tissue regeneration. Int Periodontol Restor Dent 1988; 4.

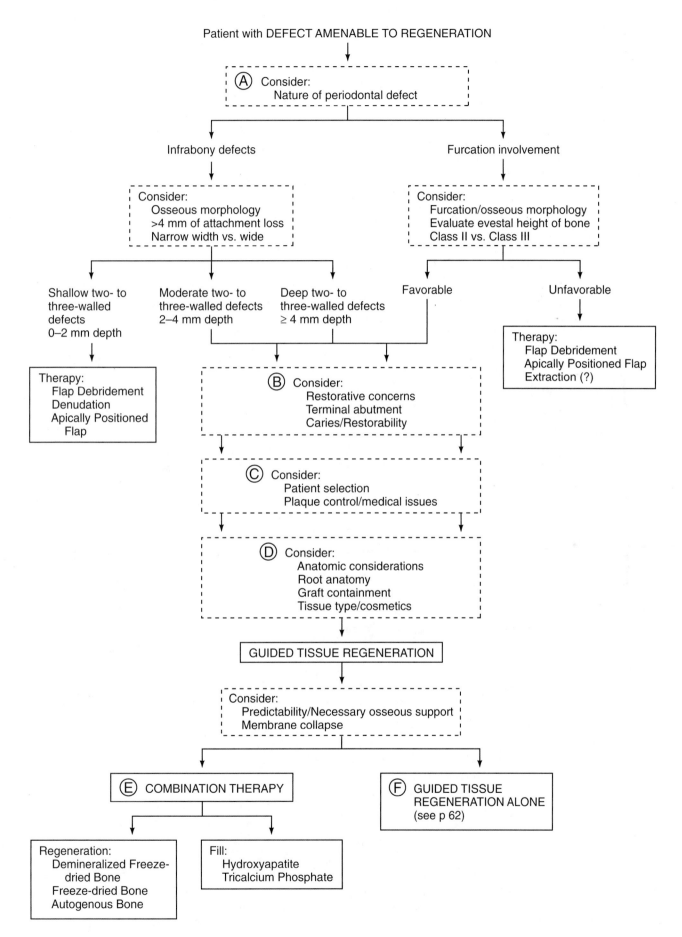

Patient with DEFECT AMENABLE TO REGENERATION

A Consider:
　Nature of periodontal defect

Infrabony defects

Consider:
　Osseous morphology
　>4 mm of attachment loss
　Narrow width vs. wide

Shallow two- to three-walled defects 0–2 mm depth

Moderate two- to three-walled defects 2–4 mm depth

Deep two- to three-walled defects ≥ 4 mm depth

Therapy:
　Flap Debridement
　Denudation
　Apically Positioned Flap

B Consider:
　Restorative concerns
　Terminal abutment
　Caries/Restorability

C Consider:
　Patient selection
　Plaque control/medical issues

D Consider:
　Anatomic considerations
　Root anatomy
　Graft containment
　Tissue type/cosmetics

GUIDED TISSUE REGENERATION

Consider:
　Predictability/Necessary osseous support
　Membrane collapse

E COMBINATION THERAPY

Regeneration:
　Demineralized Freeze-dried Bone
　Freeze-dried Bone
　Autogenous Bone

Fill:
　Hydroxyapatite
　Tricalcium Phosphate

F GUIDED TISSUE REGENERATION ALONE
(see p 62)

Furcation involvement

Consider:
　Furcation/osseous morphology
　Evaluate evestal height of bone
　Class II vs. Class III

Favorable

Unfavorable

Therapy:
　Flap Debridement
　Apically Positioned Flap
　Extraction (?)

57

FURCATION INVOLVEMENTS

Walter B. Hall

The type and severity of furcation involvements on molar teeth represent a critical concern in treatment planning for a patient with a complex dental problem. Furcation involvements are categorized as follows: Class I, incipient; Class II, definite; or Class III, through and through (Fig. 1).

Each furcation should be explored with a pig-tailed type of explorer or "furca finder." Insert the instrument into the furca and move it laterally and coronally to determine whether the instrument can slip out. The type of furcation involvement is recorded on the chart, and the options for its treatment are then considered.

A. An incipient (Class I) furca exists when the instrument slips out of the furca when moved anteriorly, posteriorly, or coronally or in proximal furcas when moved facially, lingually, and coronally. It is recorded with the symbol "∧" placed appropriately on the tooth diagram. Such furcas are unlikely to influence the treatment plan but should be documented. If the incipient involvement is a deep one that does not produce a definite catch because adjacent roots are fused, guided tissue regeneration (see p 62) should be considered.

B. A definite (Class II) furca exists when a definite catch prevents removal of the furca finder coronally or laterally but definitely stops before going "through and through" to another furca opening. It is recorded with the symbol "△" placed in the appropriate furca on the

tooth diagram. The severity of the involvement horizontally determines the best treatment option. If the furca finder can be advanced less than 3 mm horizontally into the defect, osseous resection and pocket elimination represent a good treatment option. If the furca finder can be advanced 3 mm or more into the defect, guided tissue regeneration is a predictable approach for regaining lost attachment and creating a maintainable situation. Often the horizontal measurement is recorded in millimeters apical to the symbol of the chart.

C. A through and through (Class III) furca exists when the furca finder is inserted and appears to connect directly with one or more other furcas. It is recorded by placing the symbol "▲" in each of the appropriate furca areas on the tooth diagram; therefore, more than one "▲" symbol must be used on a tooth to document a Class III situation. If a tooth with a class III furca is not critical to the overall treatment plan, it should be extracted. If its retention does not jeopardize the overall treatment plan, it may be maintained (guided tissue regeneration may become a predictable treatment for such teeth in the near future). If the tooth is a critical one and its retention in a maintainable and useful manner can be achieved by hemisection or root amputation, such an approach, although expensive, often can significantly improve the overall treatment plan for a complex case.

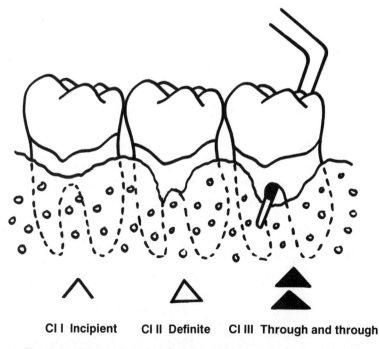

CI I Incipient   CI II Definite   CI III Through and through

Figure 1. Classes of symbols and appearance of furcation involvements.

Patient with a COMPLEX DENTAL PROBLEM AND A MOLAR WITH A FURCATION INVOLVEMENT

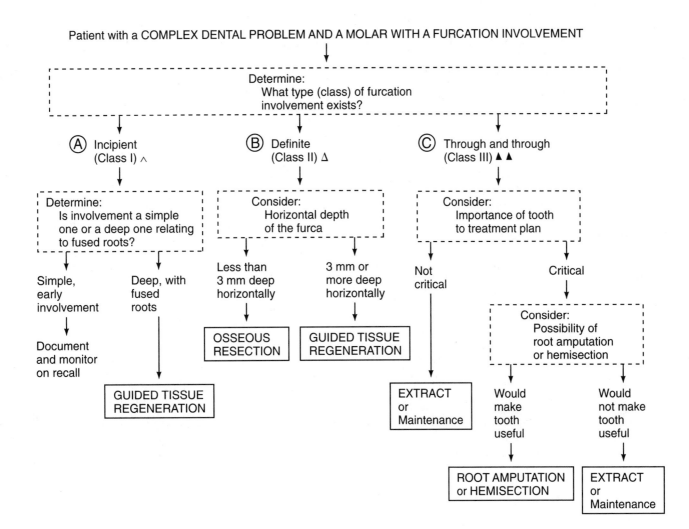

References

Carranza FA. Clinical periodontology. 7th ed. Philadelphia: WB Saunders, 1990:259, 494, 860.
Easley JF, Drennan GA. Morphological classification of the furca. J Can Dent Assoc 1969; 3512.
Genco RJ, Goldman HM, Cohen DW. Contemporary periodontics. St Louis: CV Mosby, 1990:344, 354.

Grant DA, Stern JB, Listgarten MA. Periodontics. 6th ed. St Louis: CV Mosby, 1988:921.
Heins PJ, Carter SR: Furca involvement: A classification of bony deformities. Periodontics 1968; 6:84.
Schluger S, Yuodelis R, Page RC, Johnson RH. Periodontal diseases. 2nd ed. Philadelphia: Lea & Febiger, 1990:545.
Tarnow D, Fletcher P. Classification of the vertical component of furcation involvement. J Periodontol 1984; 55:283.-

EVALUATION OF FURCATION STATUS OF MOLARS BEFORE SURGERY

Walter B. Hall

When initial therapy evaluation is performed several weeks or more following root planing and any other aspects of initial treatment, the status of furcation involvements of molar teeth becomes an important consideration in deciding whether surgery would be beneficial to the patient. If furcations are readily accessible for plaque removal and root planing, maintenance by regular root planing several times a year is a reasonable option for controlling progress of inflammatory periodontal disease. If the furcations are not accessible for plaque removal and root planing, surgery may make them accessible and improve the prognosis for the tooth. An individual molar should be treated on the basis of the worst furcation involvement present (Fig. 1).

A. The type of furcation involvement must be assessed when determining treatment options. If furcations are not involved, maintenance by root planing alone usually is a good option. The status of adjacent teeth and pocket depths on the individual molar may make surgery a desirable option in some cases, even when furcations are not involved. Class I (incipient) and Class II (definite) involvements require considerable decision making. Class III (through and through) involvements are not treatable predictably for regeneration. Mandibular molars have two furcations that must be evaluated in deciding on further therapy at the time of initial therapy evaluation; maxillary molars have three furcations.

B. If the worst involvement is incipient (Class I), maintenance with regular root planing several times a year usually suffices. If the roots are fused, a Class I furcation may be all that is present to the apex of the tooth, in which case pocket depths and type of osseous defect present become critical factors. If pocket depth is slight, the tooth may be maintained; however, if it is extensive, guided tissue regeneration (GTR) with the expectation of regaining lost attachment may be possible. Most defects associated with fused roots have three osseous walls, making them good candidates for GTR. Should the roots be tortuous and the defect not accessible to instrumentation surgically, the tooth should be extracted or maintained with a hopeless prognosis.

C. If the molar has a Class II (definite) involvement, access for plaque removal and root planing is a most important consideration in deciding on the value of surgery. Because maxillary molars have proximal furcations, access is a greater problem in that arch than in mandibular molars. If access is good, maintenance with regular root planing several times a year may be sufficient. The status of adjacent teeth may make inclusion of molars with Class II furcations in surgery a desirable option even though they are accessible for maintenance. If the access is not good, so that adequate plaque removal and root planing are difficult or impossible to accomplish, loss of attachment and type of osseous defect present become the chief factors in deciding on treatment. If the defect is less than 3 mm straight in, mucogingival-osseous surgery with an apically positioned flap approach makes the area accessible for instrumentation and plaque removal. If the defect is 3 mm or more straight in, a three-walled osseous defect usually is present on facial or lingual furcas; proximal furcas can have two- or three-walled defects. All are good candidates for GTR.

D. Class III, through and through, furcas are not amenable to predictable GTR as yet.

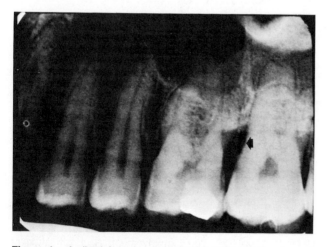

Figure 1. A distal furcation involvement on the first molar with apparent second molar root proximity.

References

Carranza FA. Clinical periodontology. 7th ed. Philadelphia: WB Saunders, 1990:860.

Genco RJ, Goldman HM, Cohen DW. Contemporary periodontics. St Louis: CV Mosby, 1990:344, 354, 409.

Hemp SE, Nyman S, Lindhe J. Treatment of multi-rooted teeth. Results after 5 years. J Clin Periodontol 1975; 2:126.

Lindhe J. Textbook of clinical periodontology. 2nd ed. Copenhagen: Munksgaard, 1989:515.

Schluger S, Yuodelis R, Page RC, Johnson RH. Periodontal diseases. 2nd ed. Philadelphia: Lea & Febiger, 1990:541.

Patient for INITIAL THERAPY EVALUATION OF A MOLAR TOOTH

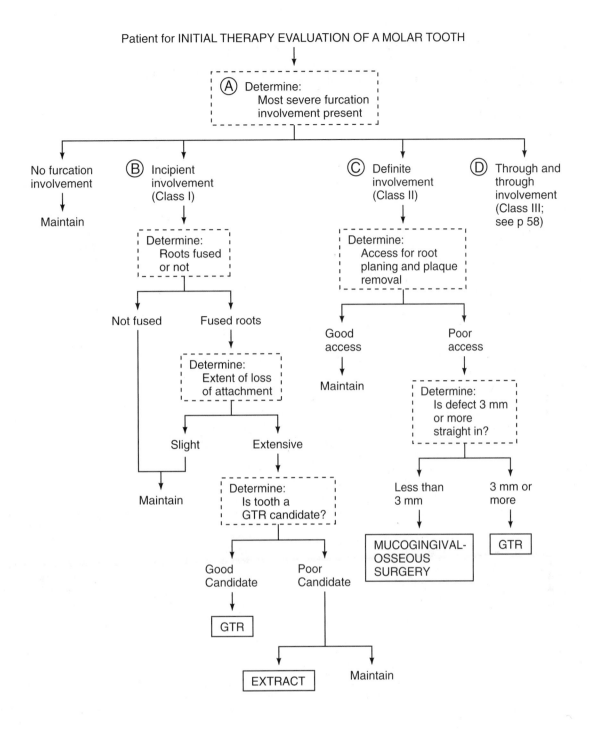

GUIDED TISSUE REGENERATION OR ALTERNATIVES FOR TREATING FURCATION INVOLVEMENTS

Jon Zabelegui
Alberto Sicilia

One of the most common difficulties encountered in treating periodontal disease is the presence of a furcation involvement. The ultimate goal of periodontal therapy is the regeneration of the periodontium to a state of health and function. Historically, with furcation involvement treatment and prognosis have been difficult. Results with conventional therapy are unpredictable, but guided tissue regeneration (GTR) in some furcations consistently has been reported to be predictable if certain characteristics are found.

A. A furcation involvement exists when attachment exposes the furcation to probing. Depending on how much attachment has been lost, it can be classified as Class I, II, or III. Furcation involvements are a periodontal hazard because they are difficult to clean even by professional means. Class I furcations are those where the tip of the probe does not catch within the furcation. This situation is easy to control; mild modification of the contour (odontoplasty) of the crown with a cylindrical finishing bur allows the tooth to be cleaned.

B. When the probe catches in the furcation when moved coronally or in either lateral direction, a Class II or Class III furcation involvement is present. If an instrument goes into one furcation and comes out of another, a through and through or Class III furcation involvement is present; if it cannot do so, a definite or Class II furcation involvement is present.

C. With Class II or III furcation involvement, a decision whether GTR or resective surgery should be performed is based on the apical depth of the furca involvement in relation to the bone levels between the involved molar and adjacent teeth. This may be assessed radiographically and by probing.

D. If the furcation pocket depth is deep to that of the crestal bone between the involved tooth and its adjacent neighbors, GTR should be considered; however, if root proximity (p 68) limits access for debridement (e.g., there is only a narrow opening), resective surgery is a better option unless the roots are fused.

  In some GTR situations, bone grafting to fill out a space into which regeneration tissue can grow (and prevent collapse of the membrane into the defect) may be helpful or a coronal placement of the flap may be useful.

E. If the furcation pocket depth is more shallow than the level of the crestal bone between the involved tooth and its adjacent neighbors, options include resective surgery (p 54), hemisection or root amputation, (p 128), or extraction (p 8).

References

Anderegg OR, Martin SJ, Gray JL, et al. Clinical evaluation of the use of decalcified freeze-dried bone allograft with guided tissue regeneration in the treatment of molar furcation invasions. J Periodontol 1991; 62:264.

Becker W, Becker B, Berg L, et al. New attachment after treatment with root isolation procedures: Report for treated Class III and Class II furcations and vertical osseous defects. Int J Periodontol Restor Dent 1988; 3(3):9.

Carranza FA. Clinical periodontology. 7th ed. Philadelphia: WB Saunders, 1990:547, 841.

Gottlow J, Nyman S, Karring T, Wennstrom J. New attachment formation in human periodontium by guided tissue regeneration. 1986; 57:727.

Pontoriero R, Lindhe J, Nyman S, et al. Guided tissue regeneration in degree II furcation involved mandibular teeth. J Clin Periodontol 1988; 15:247.

Patient with a COMPLEX DENTAL PROBLEM AND A MOLAR WITH A FURCATION INVOLVEMENT

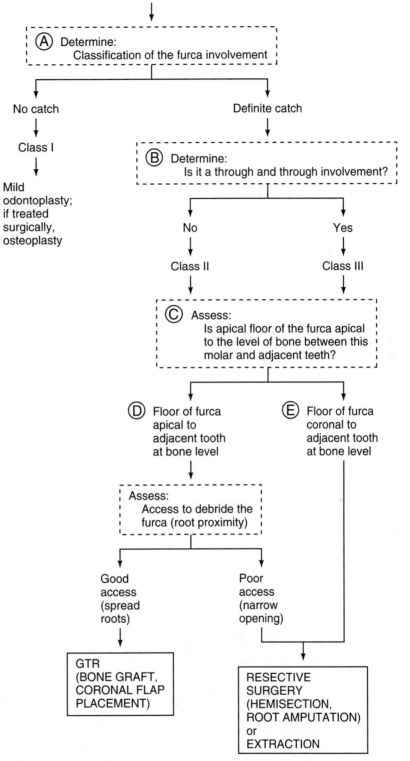

A Determine:
  Classification of the furca involvement

No catch

Class I

Mild
odontoplasty;
if treated
surgically,
osteoplasty

Definite catch

B Determine:
  Is it a through and through involvement?

No

Class II

Yes

Class III

C Assess:
  Is apical floor of the furca apical
  to the level of bone between this
  molar and adjacent teeth?

D Floor of furca
  apical to
  adjacent tooth
  at bone level

E Floor of furca
  coronal to
  adjacent tooth
  at bone level

Assess:
  Access to debride the
  furca (root proximity)

Good
access
(spread
roots)

Poor
access
(narrow
opening)

GTR
(BONE GRAFT,
CORONAL FLAP
PLACEMENT)

RESECTIVE
SURGERY
(HEMISECTION,
ROOT AMPUTATION)
or
EXTRACTION

MANAGEMENT OF A THREE-WALLED OSSEOUS DEFECT ON AN ABUTMENT TOOTH

Walter B. Hall

A three-walled osseous defect on an abutment tooth offers significant opportunities for treatment that can "make or break" a treatment plan in a complex case. The opportunities for regaining lost attachment have improved impressively with the development of guided tissue regeneration. Implants offer opportunities that were not predictable 5 to 10 years ago. The dentist has an obligation to discuss these possibilities with the patient and to select a treatment that best meets the patient's individual objectives and means.

A. The severity of the three-walled defect (Fig. 1) affects which options offer the most predictable results for the patient. A shallow-walled defect (1 to 2 mm in depth) often is best managed with pocket elimination mucogingival-osseous surgery when the defect can be eliminated without affecting the utility of the tooth as an abutment or with respect to esthetic demands while improving access for plaque removal and recall root planing. If esthetics would be compromised, the defect is very shallow, or surgery can or should be avoided for health or personal reasons, maintenance care may suffice.

B. If the defect is 3 mm or greater in depth but is narrow (1 mm or less measured horizontally from root to crest of bone), it is amenable to osseous fill with new attachment by the method of Prichard in which complete debridement of the narrow defect results in the formation of new bone and creation of a new connective tissue attachment filling the defect.

C. If the defect is 3 mm or more in depth and is wider than 1 mm from root to osseous crest measured horizontally, a Prichard approach would only result in fill in the narrower, deeper portion with a residual defect remaining. Guided tissue regeneration using a GoreTex barrier (see p 66) predictably results in a new attachment regenerating from the ligament, often with significant new bone formation (Fig. 2). Neither the extremity of the depth of the defect nor the presence of a furcation involvement (as long as it is not through and through, Class III), makes this approach less predictable. A potential abutment thus involved had little chance of being usable prior to the development of guided tissue regeneration. Now this approach is the treatment of choice if the tooth is a critical one. If it is not a critical abutment, it could be extracted. If guided tissue regeneration fails, an implant may be considered. As guided tissue regeneration is a more predictable procedure than a single tooth implant and is far less expensive, it should be employed prior to considering an implant.

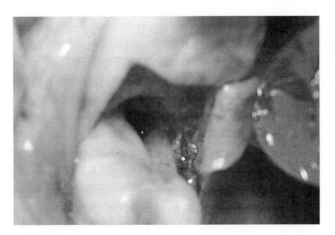

Figure 1.   A deep, wide three-walled osseous defect on a critical abutment tooth exposed for guided tissue regeneration.

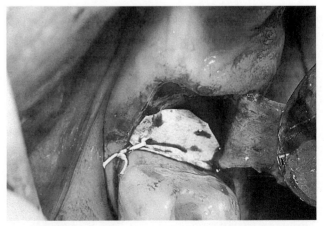

Figure 2.   A GoreTex membrane has been sutured and covers the debrided defect.

Patient with a COMPLEX DENTAL PROBLEM AND A THREE-WALLED DEFECT ON AN ABUTMENT

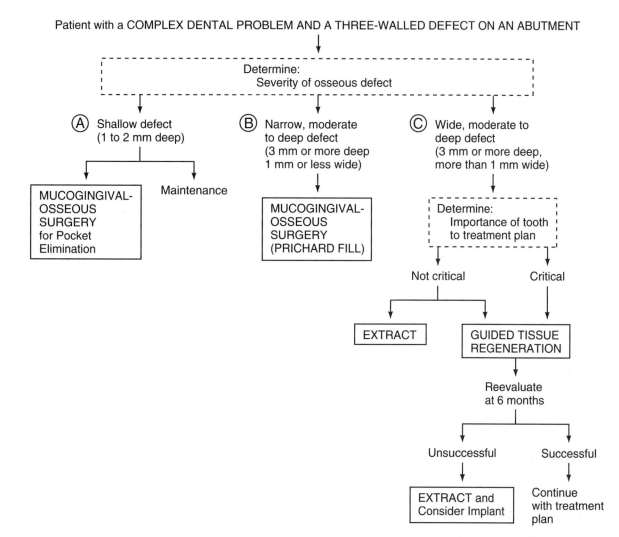

References

Bowers GM, Schallhorn RG, Mellonig JR. Histologic evaluation of new attachment in human intrabony defects. A literature review. J Periodontol 1982; 53:509.

Carranza FA. Clinical periodontology. 7th ed. Philadelphia: WB Saunders, 1990:836.

Caton J, Nyman S, Zander H. Histometric evaluation of periodontal surgery. II. Connective tissue attachment levels after four regenerative procedures. J Clin Periodontol 1980; 7:224.

Prichard JF. The infrabony technique as a predictable procedure. J Periodontol 1957; 28:202.

Prichard JF. A technique for treating intrabony pockets based on alveolar process morphology. Dent Clin North Am 1960; 3:85.

Schallhorn RG, Hiatt WH. Human allografts of iliac cancellous bone and marrow in periodontal osseous defects. II. Clinical observations. J Periodontol 1972; 43:67.

GUIDED TISSUE REGENERATION IN THREE-WALLED OSSEOUS DEFECTS

Jon Zabelegui
Alberto Sicilia

Of all the bone defects created by periodontal disease, the three-walled defect has the highest predictability of successful regeneration. A three-walled defect is delimited by three bony walls: buccal, mesial or distal, and lingual. The fourth wall is always the surface of the root of the tooth. Radiographic examination and periodontal probing help to diagnose a three-walled defect; two different osseous levels at the same site—one parallel to the pattern of bone level and the other aiming towards the apex of the root—suggest a three-walled defect. Probings on a possible three-walled defect are shallow at the line angles and deep in the interproximal area under the contact.

A. If the defect is shallow (1 or 2 mm deep) and wide, possible approaches include an apically positioned flap with osseous recontouring of the architecture or an open flap debridement.

B. If the defect is deep and wide with deep surrounding vestibular depth, perform guided tissue regeneration (GTR). Choose the wraparound configuration that best covers the defect, overlapping 2 to 3 mm over the osseous walls. An autograft or allograft of autogenous bone is sometimes used. Denudation with secondary intention healing may be useful with narrow defects.

C. If the defect is deep with shallow surrounding vestibular depth, perform GTR. Choose the wraparound configuration that best covers the defect, overlapping 2 to 3 mm over the osseous walls. An autograft or allograft of autogenous bone may be used so that the gingival tissue does not push the GTR membrane into the defect (which would not allow enough space for the regenerative tissue to form). Denudation with secondary intention healing is a less satisfactory alternative. Extraction of the tooth may be necessary if the restorative plan is extensive and the prognosis of the tooth cannot be improved by other treatment methods. Extraction may be necessary if the three-walled defect totally surrounds the four surfaces of the tooth and trauma from occlusion cannot be controlled.

The most critical factor in obtaining maximum results with GTR is the availability of good access for root debridement. Collapse of the periodontal membrane used into the defect must be avoided by properly managing the sutures and surrounding (hard and soft) tissues to membrane relationships. The flap should be elevated so that no tension occurs at the time of closure; either vertical releasing incisions and/or extending two teeth aside of the treated area is recommended for this purpose.

References

Becker W, Becker B, Berg L, et al. New attachment after treatment with root isolation procedures: Report for treated Class III and Class II furcations and vertical defects. Int J Periodont Restorat Dent 1988; 8(3):9.

Becker W, Becker B, Berg L, Sansom O. Clinical and volumetric analysis of three-walled intrabony defects following open flap debridement. J Periodontol 1986; 57:277.

Carranza FA. Clinical periodontology. 7th ed. Philadelphia, WB Saunders, 1990:546, 841.

Gottlow J, Nyman S, Karring T, Wennstrom J. New attachment formation in human periodontium by guided tissue regeneration. J Periodontol 1986; 57:727.

Schallhorn RC, McClain PR. Combined osseous composite grafting, root conditioning and guided tissue regeneration. Int J Periodontol Restor Dent 1988; 8(4):9.

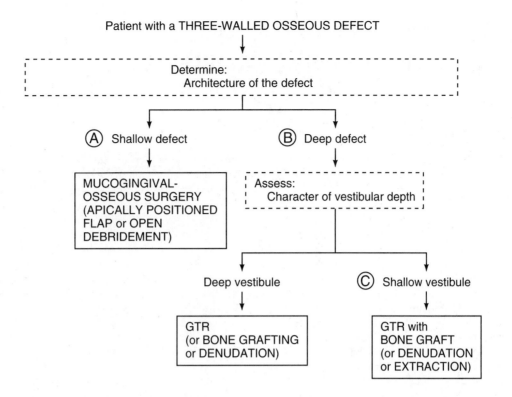

Patient with a THREE-WALLED OSSEOUS DEFECT

Determine:
Architecture of the defect

Ⓐ Shallow defect

Ⓑ Deep defect

MUCOGINGIVAL-
OSSEOUS SURGERY
(APICALLY POSITIONED
FLAP or OPEN
DEBRIDEMENT)

Assess:
Character of vestibular depth

Deep vestibule

Ⓒ Shallow vestibule

GTR
(or BONE GRAFTING
or DENUDATION)

GTR with
BONE GRAFT
(or DENUDATION
or EXTRACTION)

MAXILLARY MOLARS WITH ROOT PROXIMITY/PERIODONTAL PROBLEMS

Walter B. Hall

Maxillary molar teeth with periodontal problems complicated by root proximity (roots so close together that plaque removal and root planing cannot be accomplished because plaque removal devices and curettes cannot be manipulated in the available space) are a common treatment planning puzzle. A surgical procedure that would eliminate pocketing but leave an area where plaque removal by the patient and root planing by the therapist cannot be performed effectively is not a wise choice for therapy. Extraction of or root amputation on one or both of the molars can create a sound, maintainable, functional unit but involves extensive treatment including endodontics and/or prosthodontics as well as periodontal treatment. Such treatment is expensive and must be within the patient's means. Guided tissue regeneration (GTR) is not feasible if root proximity negates the possibility of thorough debridement of the periodontal defect; however, if the area can be thoroughly debrided, guided tissue regeneration could be an effective and comparatively inexpensive approach. See Fig. 1.

A. If the defect between the two molars can be thoroughly debrided with a curette following flap displacement, guided tissue regeneration is the best option.

B. If GTR is not feasible, the endodontic status of the two molars should be determined next. If no pulpal problem exists, a determination should be made whether root canal therapy and a root amputation can be done. If so, the restorability of the teeth and their value to the overall treatment plan should be assessed. If restoration is feasible and useful and the periodontal problem can be resolved by root amputation on either or both of the molars (and the patient consents to and can afford this approach), endodontics followed by root amputation/periodontal surgical therapy should be performed and the teeth restored appropriately. If root canal therapy or root amputation cannot be done (e.g., root tips are fused) or if the restorative and periodontal problems cannot be resolved by root amputation, either or both of the molars may have to be extracted and the problem resolved prosthodontically or with implants.

C. If either or both of the molars also have endodontic problems, the possibility of performing successful root canal therapy should be evaluated first. If they can be treated, the sequence of decision making would be the same as in B: (1) Can a root amputation be done?

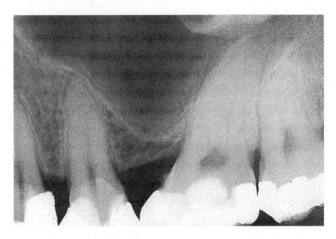

Figure 1. Root proximity between second and third molars appears to jeopardize access to successfully treat or maintain the distal furcation involvement on the second molar.

(2) Can the periodontal problem be resolved and the teeth restored to usefulness in the overall treatment plan? (3) Can the patient accept and afford this approach?

If the answer to each question is positive, proceed with endodontics, root amputation/periodontal surgery, and restoration. If the answer to any of the questions is negative, extraction of one or both molars and a prosthodontic or implant solution should be considered.

D. If one or both of the molars have existing endodontics, the adequacy of the existing endodontics (including "cracked tooth" signs or symptoms) should be evaluated first. If the endodontics is satisfactory and no vertical root fractures can be detected, the sequence of decision making would be the same as in C. If the answer to each question is positive and no endodontic retreatment is needed, root amputation and elimination of the periodontal defects should be performed and followed by appropriate restoration. If the answer to each question is positive and the existing endodontics is unsatisfactory but it can be redone successfully or the problem is around the root to be amputated, necessary endodontic retreatment followed by root amputation/periodontal surgery and restoration should be planned. If any answers are negative, extraction and a prosthodontic or implant alternative should be employed.

Patient with MAXILLARY MOLARS WITH ROOT PROXIMITY/PERIODONTAL PROBLEMS

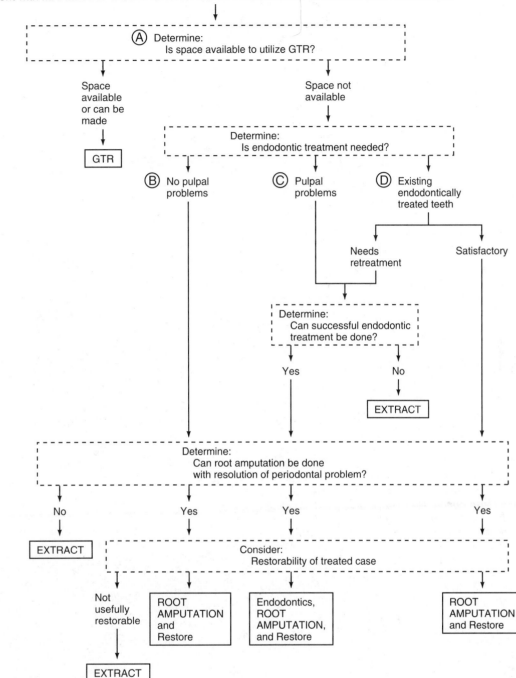

References

Carranza FA. Clinical periodontology. 7th ed. Philadelphia: WB Saunders, 1990:867.

Genco RJ, Goldman HM, Cohen DW. Contemporary periodontics. St Louis: CV Mosby, 1990:582, 589.

Hall WB. Periodontal preparation of the mouth for restoration. Dent Clin North Am 1980; 24:197.

Hall WB. Removal of third molars. A periodontal viewpoint. In: McDonald RE, Hurt WC, Gilmore HW, Middleton RH, eds. Current therapy in dentistry. St Louis: CV Mosby, 1980:228.

Schluger S, Yuodelis R, Page RC, Johnson RH. Periodontal diseases. 2nd ed. Philadelphia: Lea & Febiger, 1990:102, 343, 511.

GUIDED TISSUE REGENERATION IN TWO-WALLED OSSEOUS DEFECTS

Alberto Sicilia
Jon Zabelegui
Jose Maria Tejerina

Although a two-walled osseous defect frequently can be diagnosed through careful clinical and radiographic examination or with sounding, in many cases its presence and morphology up to the moment of the surgical debridement of the defect are not certain. For this reason the approach must be carried out through a full thickness flap to determine whether guided tissue regeneration (GTR) is indirected.

A. In shallow defects regeneration is difficult to achieve or very little regeneration results. When the cost-benefit relationship compared with other kinds of treatment is unfavorable, GTR is not recommended.

B. In very deep defects the prognosis of the adjacent tooth or teeth must be evaluated. If hopeless (see p 8), GTR should not be performed.

C. In moderate defects or in deep ones that are treatable, GTR must be considered. Its application requires an adequate separation of the roots of the adjacent teeth. When less than 2 mm is present, application of the technique is unlikely to be useful.

D. When the separation between adjacent teeth is adequate, the anatomy of the defect and adjacent teeth determines whether GTR is appropriate. If it is possible to totally close the entrance of the defect and create a free space underneath the membrane itself, GTR is an option. If the membrane does not totally close the entrance of the defect (e.g., in the case of a very big entrance defect or a tooth with marked concavity on its affected surface) or it collapses against the wall of the defect (e.g., in the case of a defect where the walls do not adequately support the membrane in the right position), GTR would not be appropriate (Fig. 1). The amount of healthy periodontium close to the defect is also important; narrow and deep defects are more favorable than those that are wide and shallow (Fig. 2).

E. A thick periodontium and an adequate vestibule facilitate the viability and stability of the flap that covers the membrane; this reduces the risk of plaque accumulation over it, which can jeopardize regeneration. The absence of adequate gingiva can also compromise the success of GTR.

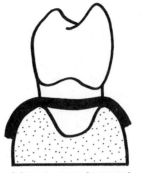
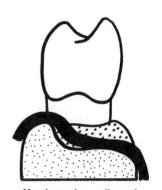

Adequate space is created　　**Membrane has collapsed**

FAVORABLE SITUATION　　**UNFAVORABLE SITUATION**

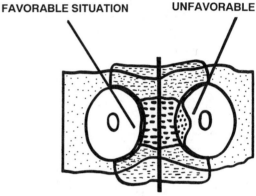

Well adapted membrane　　**Badly adapted membrane**

Figure 1. Favorable versus unfavorable situations to prevent membrane collapse.

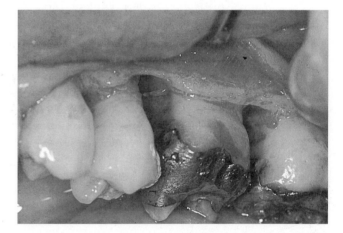

Figure 2. Typical deep two-walled infrabony craters between second premolar and first molar and between first and second molars are good candidates for GTR.

Patient with a COMPLEX PROBLEM AND A TWO-WALLED OSSEOUS DEFECT

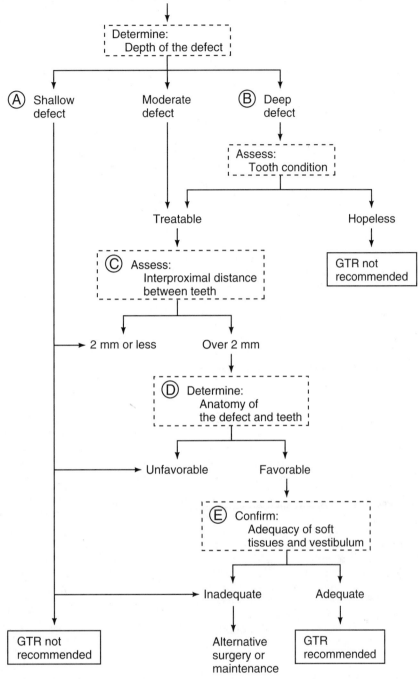

References

Becker W, Becker BE, Berg L, et al. New attachment after treatment with root isolation procedures: Report for treated class II furcations and vertical osseous defects. Int

J Periodontol Restor Dent 1988; 3:2.
Carranza FA Jr. Clinical periodontology. 7th ed. Philadelphia: WB Saunders, 1990:836.
World Workshop in Clinical Periodontics. Chicago: American Academy of Periodontology, 1989.

GUIDED TISSUE REGENERATION VERSUS IMPLANTS

William P. Lundergan

Rapid progress in the field of implantology and the development of guided tissue regeneration (GTR) were among the many advances in the 1990s. In the 1990s, the dentist must consider these treatment alternatives when confronted with a periodontally compromised tooth. Should the tooth be treated using GTR or should it be extracted and replaced with an implant? Choosing between these two procedures or an alternative therapy requires careful consideration.

A. The nature of the periodontal bony defect is very important when assessing the prospects for success with GTR. The procedure is not successful in treating areas of horizontal bone loss as the membrane will be unable to maintain a space in which regeneration can occur. Consider GTR in treating two- and three-walled vertical defects and Class II furcation involvements. Success in treating one-walled vertical defects and Class III furcation involvements is less predictable. Consider implant therapy if GTR procedures are unlikely to be successful.

B. The anatomy of the tooth in question must be evaluated when considering GTR. Root concavities and furcation involvement can complicate the procedure as complete adaptation of the open microstructure portion of the membrane to the tooth is critical. If the membrane is poorly adapted, epithelial cells are able to migrate apically along the root surface and prevent regeneration. Thus, when treating a tooth with furcation involvement, a long root trunk is preferred to a short root trunk as the chances of successfully adapting the membrane are enhanced. The clinician must also consider the potential postsurgical maintenance problems created by root concavities, grooves, and furcation exposure. Root morphology and length should also be evaluated. If the tooth is eventually to serve as an abutment, will the periodontal support be adequate even if GTR is successful? All these factors must be considered.

C. Prior to performing GTR the ultimate restorability of the tooth should be evaluated. If the tooth is fractured, perforated, or internally/externally resorbed, can these complicating factors be satisfactorily resolved? If the tooth requires endodontic therapy, what are the prospects for successful treatment? If the roots are severely dilacerated or the canals calcified, the chance for success may not be very good. The position of the tooth in the arch should also be considered from the standpoints of strategic location and maintainability. If the tooth is not in a favorable position, is orthodontic therapy indicated and what are the prospects for success? If esthetic concerns are involved, can the tooth be restored with an acceptable esthetic result? Finally, the decision must consider the overall treatment plan for the patient. Is GTR compatible with the overall treatment plan, or would extraction be more appropriate?

D. GTR procedures are not recommended for patients with heart valve defects, prosthetic devices, uncontrolled diabetes, or immune defects. Any factor that contraindicates periodontal surgery also contraindicates GTR; in such cases an alternative therapy should be considered.

E. The dentist must consider several factors when planning the surgical placement of an implant. Anatomic considerations include the type of bone present, available vertical bone height, buccolingual width of the alveolar ridge, maxillary sinus location, mandibular nerve location, and surgical access. Some potentially limiting anatomic factors can be corrected using advanced surgical techniques (e.g., sinus lift, mandibular nerve repositioning procedure) but not without increased cost and risk of complications. Alveolar ridge deficiencies may be corrected using ridge augmentation procedures (i.e., bone grafting and/or GTR). Medical contraindications for the surgical placement of implants might include recent myocardial infarction, poorly controlled diabetes, immunosuppression, head and neck radiation therapy, risk for endocarditis, alcohol/drug dependency, and mental health status. The dentist must also consider patient acceptance of the overall surgical and prosthetic treatment plan including factors such as time, cost, and risk. Any single factor may make implant therapy inappropriate and require consideration of an alternative treatment plan.

F. The dentist must evaluate several prosthetic considerations when considering a dental implant: temporomandibular joint status, maxillary/mandibular ridge relationship, available interarch distance, the existence of parafunctional habits, the occlusal relationship of the remaining teeth, the patient's oral hygiene/motivation, and the patient's esthetic requirements. Any single factor may make implant therapy inappropriate and require consideration of an alternative treatment plan.

References

Bahat O. Surgical planning. J Calif Dent Assoc 1992; 20(5):31.

Carranza FA Jr. Glickman's Clinical periodontology. Philadelphia: WB Saunders, 1990:841, 956.

deGennaro G. Addressing the options. J Calif Dent Assoc 1992; 20(5):48.

Patient with a COMPLEX DENTAL PROBLEM INVOLVING A TOOTH REQUIRING
GUIDED TISSUE REGENERATION OR AN IMPLANT

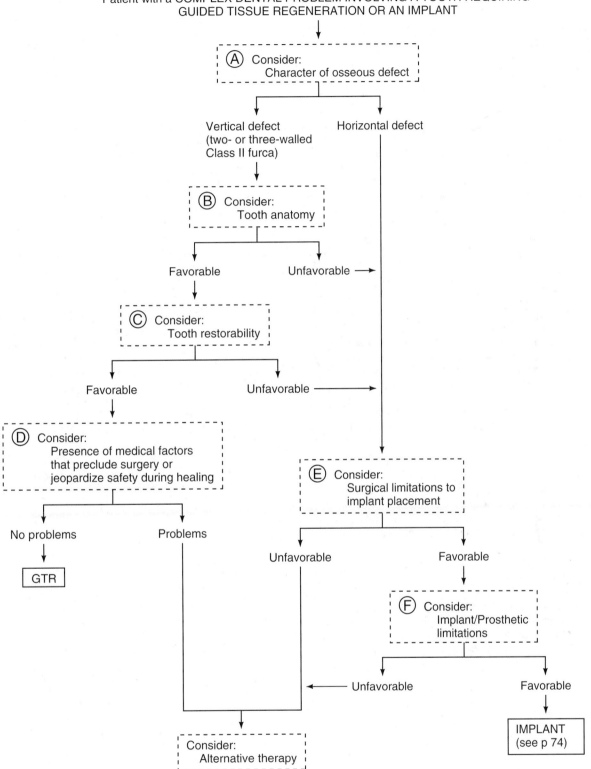

BASIC CONSIDERATIONS IN SELECTING A PATIENT FOR IMPLANTS

E. Robert Stultz, Jr.

When a patient is considering an implant approach to his edentulous or partially dentulous status, he may seek information from his general dentist or a specialist. In each case a series of decisions is made to determine whether the patient is a reasonable candidate for implant therapy. The initial decisions involve medical and psychologic qualification for implant therapy. Once these considerations are met successfully, the dental indications and contraindications can be evaluated.

A. A medical evaluation is made from a questionnaire, a patient interview, and any medical consultations necessitated by the history. Conditions that make surgery dangerous or adversely affect healing must be considered. Examples of absolute contraindications are recurrent myocardial infarction, acquired immunodeficiency virus (AIDS), debilitating or transmissible hepatitis, pregnancy, granulocytopenia, poorly controlled diabetes, and drug or alcohol dependency. Other conditions (e.g., prolonged corticosteroid use, blood dyscrasias, collagen diseases, malignancies, heavy smoking) make implant a questionable alternative. If any significant medical contraindication exists and cannot be resolved promptly, implants are not indicated and alternative approaches are required.

B. If no medical contraindications are detected, the psychologic status of the patient and the reasonableness of his expectations are evaluated. If the patient is psychologically unstable or his expectations of implant therapy are unrealistic, alternative approaches should be considered.

C. If the patient is psychologically well adjusted and does not expect "miracles" in esthetics or functional benefits of an implant approach, the consequences of his totally edentulous or partially dentulous status should be considered next. The status of teeth to be retained are a complicating factor in this decision process. Position of these teeth, their periodontal status, and their restorability must be considered.

D. To determine whether adequate support exists for implants, the quantity of bone available at implant sites must be evaluated. If the height or width of the recipient ridge areas is inadequate or if the trajectory is unsatisfactory, an implant may not be feasible. Bony undercuts also present problems as do the position of anatomic features such as the mental foramen. These factors can be examined with simple dental radiographs, Panorex films, tomographic or cephalometric film, or computerized tomography scan imaging. If the ridge is inadequate for any reason, an implant is inappropriate and alternatives should be considered.

E. If bone "quantity" is satisfactory, bone "quality" should be considered next. The most ideal alveolar bone is the dense cortical bone of the mandibular anterior ridge; the least desirable is the thin cortical, loose trabecular bone typically found in the maxillary posterior region. Bone quality may be classified as follows:

Class I: Dense cortical bone
Class II: Dense cortical bone with dense trabecular bone
Class III: Moderate cortical and trabecular bone
Class IV: Thin cortical bone with poor trabecular bone

Patients with Class I or II bone are good candidates for osseointegrated implants. Those with Class III or IV bone require bone augmentation before osseointegrated implants or a subperiosteal approach.

References

Branemark PI, Zarb G, Albrecktesson T. Tissue integrated prosthesis: Osseointegration in clinical dentistry. Chicago: Quintessence Publishing, 1985:1.

Golec TS. Implants, what and when. Calif Dent Assoc J 1987; 15:49.

Jensen O. Site classification for the osseointegrated implant. J Prosthet Dent 1989; 61:228.

Misch C, Judy K. Classification of partially edentulous arches for implant dentistry. Int J Oral Implant 1986; 12:688.

Stambaugh R. Calif Dent Assoc J 1989; 17:31.

Patient who is EDENTULOUS OR PARTIALLY DENTULOUS PATIENT AND CONSIDERING IMPLANTS

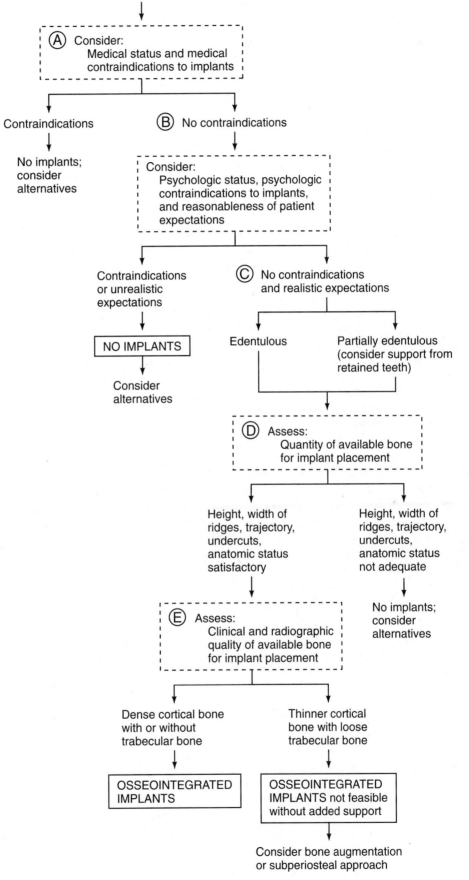

Ⓐ Consider:
Medical status and medical contraindications to implants

Contraindications

No implants; consider alternatives

Ⓑ No contraindications

Consider:
Psychologic status, psychologic contraindications to implants, and reasonableness of patient expectations

Contraindications or unrealistic expectations

NO IMPLANTS

Consider alternatives

Ⓒ No contraindications and realistic expectations

Edentulous

Partially edentulous (consider support from retained teeth)

Ⓓ Assess:
Quantity of available bone for implant placement

Height, width of ridges, trajectory, undercuts, anatomic status satisfactory

Height, width of ridges, trajectory, undercuts, anatomic status not adequate

No implants; consider alternatives

Ⓔ Assess:
Clinical and radiographic quality of available bone for implant placement

Dense cortical bone with or without trabecular bone

Thinner cortical bone with loose trabecular bone

OSSEOINTEGRATED IMPLANTS

OSSEOINTEGRATED IMPLANTS not feasible without added support

Consider bone augmentation or subperiosteal approach

SELECTION OF IMPLANT MODALITIES FOR PARTIALLY DENTULOUS PATIENTS

E. Robert Stultz, Jr.

Once the basic factors that determine the eligibility of a patient for implant therapy have been met (see p 74), the periodontal status of teeth to be retained must be determined.

A. If the remaining teeth are healthy periodontally, an implant approach to implant therapy for the partially dentulous patient becomes feasible.

B. If significant periodontal problems are detected (e.g., deep pockets, furcation involvement, poor crown to root ratio), the likelihood of treatment making affected teeth useful in the overall treatment plan must be assessed. The ability of the patient to perform adequate plaque control can be evaluated during the periodontal treatment phase. If the periodontal problems are refractory (response is poor) or good plaque control is not demonstrated, implants are not likely to be helpful and alternatives should be explored.

C. If the periodontal problems appear resolvable, their efficacy must be established following treatment. Unsuccessful cases should not receive implant therapy. Implant therapy is feasible in successful cases.

D. The available bone support is considered next. If alveolar bone height is greater than 10 mm, its width greater than 6 mm, and the trajectory less than 25 degrees, endosseous cylinder implants are the best approach.

E. If the available bone height is less than 10 mm, the width only 4 to 6 mm and/or the trajectory greater than 25 degrees, endosseous blade implants are indicated.

F. If inadequate bone height or width is present for endosseous cylinder implants, either a bone augmentation or a subperiosteal implant is the best option. If bone augmentation is selected, either a sinus elevation, or membrane-associated hard tissue grafts, or a membrane-assisted augmentation may be employed in the maxillary arch. If the procedure succeeds, the adequacy of the available bone for an endosseous cylinder implant can be reassessed. In some cases guided bone augmentation can be employed at the time of placement of a cylinder implant into an extraction socket.

References

Branemark PI, Zarb G, Albrektson T. Tissue integrated prosthesis: Osseointegration in clinical dentistry. Chicago: Quintessence Publishing, 1985:1.

Golec TS. Implants, what and when. Calif Dent Assoc J 1987; 15:49.

Jensen O. Site classification for the osseointegrated implant. J Prosthet Dent 1989; 61:228.

Misch C, Judy K. Classification of partially edentulous arches for implant dentistry. Int J Periodontol Restor Dent 1986; 12:688.

Meffert RM, Block MS, Kent JN. What is osseointegration? Int J Periodontol Restor Dent 1987; 11:135.

Smiler DG. Evaluation and treatment planning. Calif Dent Assoc J 1987; 15:35.

EVALUATING PERIODONTAL STATUS OF PATIENT WHO MEETS BASIC CRITERIA FOR IMPLANT THERAPY

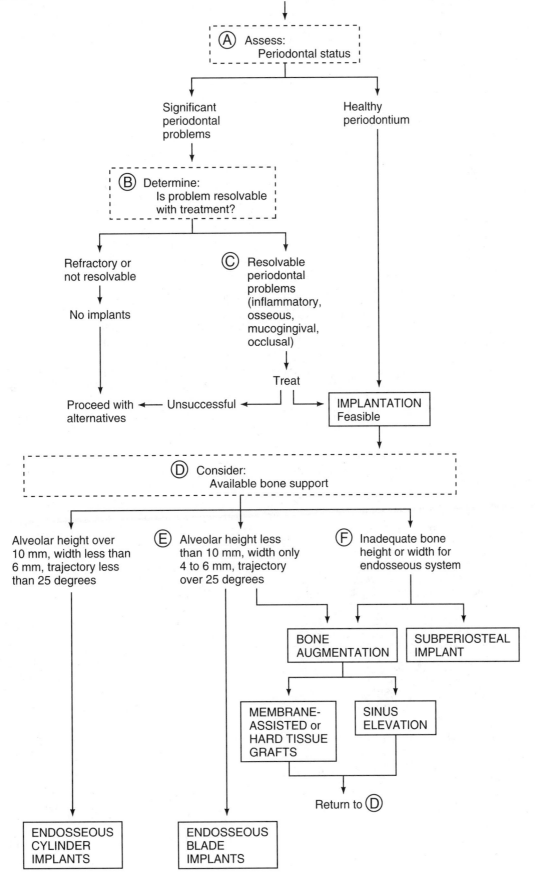

OSSEOINTEGRATED IMPLANTS FOR THE PARTIALLY EDENTULOUS MANDIBLE

Joan Pi Urgell

When the mandible is partially edentulous, three design options should be considered: Kennedy Type I (bilateral posterior edentulous areas), Type II (unilateral posterior edentulous areas), and Type III (unilateral posterior edentulous areas with anterior and posterior abutments).

A. First, investigation of the existing distance between the mandibular canal and the alveolar crest and the width of the mandibular bone is necessary. A panoramic radiograph and either conventional or computerized tomography are needed for this purpose. The radiographic study shows either that (1) the mandible is more than 8 mm high and 4 mm wide (in which case the patient is a candidate for osseointegrated implants), or (2) these necessary minimum requirements do not exist (in which case the patient is best served by a conventional prosthesis of either a fixed or removable variety). The patient's economic situation is considered in choosing the fixed (more expensive) or removable (cheaper) option.

B. In the presence of sufficient bone and absence of posterior abutment a free end saddle situation exists. The following solutions should be considered: (1) If remaining teeth need no restoration, place two implants and a free-standing bridge. (2) If the remaining teeth require restoration or root canal treatment, place one implant to support a bridge joined to the remaining teeth by means of a nonrigid anchor (a stress-broken fixed bridge).

C. When abutments remain anterior and posterior to the edentulous area (a Kennedy Type III situation) and the remaining teeth are in good condition, place two implants to support a free-standing bridge; two implants are enough for the replacement of four to six teeth if further tooth loss occurs. If the teeth are in poor condition because of extensive caries, one implant supporting a prosthesis united to the crowns of natural anterior and posterior abutments by means of semi-rigid interlocks is placed. If significant periodontal problems exist and the loss of the natural abutments might occur, one or two implants united with the natural ones by means of telescoping restorations are utilized to permit the continued use of the restoration if further tooth loss occurs.

D. When tissue-integrated prostheses cannot be considered owing to inadequate mandibular bone to allow placement of implants, conventional prostheses are the only alternative. In free end saddle cases, conventional removable prostheses are used. In cases with useful posterior abutments, a conventional fixed bridge is indicated. If the natural abutments are badly compromised periodontally and/or dentally, a conventional removable prosthesis, with or without extraction of those teeth, is the alternative.

Treatment of the partially edentulous mandible has been limited by the presence of the alveolar nerve. When there is no more than 8 mm from the mandibular canal to alveolar crest consider performing nerve lateralization to allow the fixture placement and repositioning of the alveolar nerve.

References

Ericsson I, Lekholm U, Branemark P, et al. A clinical evaluation of fixed bridge restorations supported by the combination of teeth and osseointegrated titanium implants. J Clin Periodontol 1986; 13:307.

Lekholm U. Clinical procedures for treatment with osseointegrated dental implants. J Prosthet Dent 1983; 50:1117.

Sullivan D. Prosthetic considerations for the utilization of osseointegrated fixtures in the partially edentulous arch. Int J Oral Maxillofac Implants 1986; 1:81.

Sullivan D, Krogh P. A solution of the prosthetic problem of the hemidentate arch with tissue integrated prosthesis. Int J Periodontol Restor Dent 1986; 4:66.

Patient with SOME POSTERIOR EDENTULOUS AREAS IN THE MANDIBLE

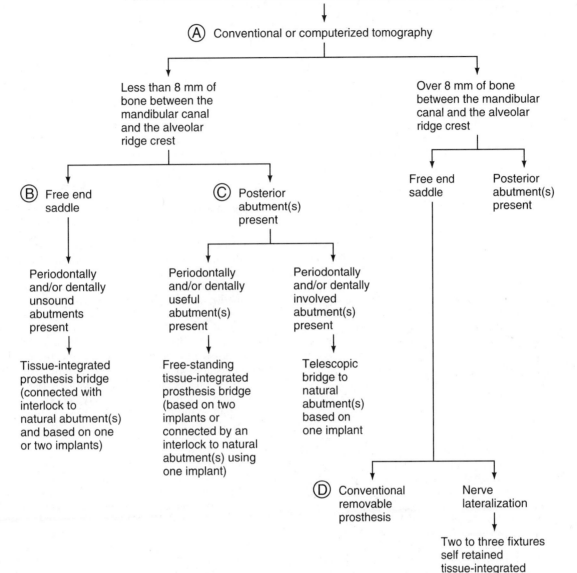

(A) Conventional or computerized tomography

Less than 8 mm of bone between the mandibular canal and the alveolar ridge crest

Over 8 mm of bone between the mandibular canal and the alveolar ridge crest

(B) Free end saddle

(C) Posterior abutment(s) present

Free end saddle

Posterior abutment(s) present

Periodontally and/or dentally unsound abutments present

Periodontally and/or dentally useful abutment(s) present

Periodontally and/or dentally involved abutment(s) present

Tissue-integrated prosthesis bridge (connected with interlock to natural abutment(s) and based on one or two implants)

Free-standing tissue-integrated prosthesis bridge (based on two implants or connected by an interlock to natural abutment(s) using one implant)

Telescopic bridge to natural abutment(s) based on one implant

(D) Conventional removable prosthesis

Nerve lateralization

Two to three fixtures self retained tissue-integrated prosthesis bridge

OSSEOINTEGRATED IMPLANTS FOR THE PARTIALLY EDENTULOUS MAXILLA

Joan Pi Urgell

When the maxilla is partially edentulous, the anatomic structures that influence the possible use of implants are the maxillary sinuses, the nasal cavity, and the surrounding bone structure. The best method of evaluating the appropriateness of these structures for the use of osseointegrated implants is computerized tomography, although conventional tomography may suffice.

A. When computerized or conventional tomography indicates lack of sufficient bone or the existence of bone of poor quality (bone that is not very trabecular), which would negate the possibility of utilizing implants, the patient is advised of the necessity of employing a conventional prosthesis. At least 8 mm of bone must be present between the maxillary sinus or nasal cavity and the crest of the alveolar ridge for osseointegrated implants to be employed.

B. If there is sufficient trabecular bone, the periodontal and dental health of the remaining teeth must be evaluated to determine the type of implant design to be employed. If the bone is of poor quality, a conventional removable prosthesis is advisable.

C. If the remaining maxillary teeth are dentally sound, their periodontal status is the determining factor in tissue-integrated prosthesis (TIP) design. Teeth that are dentally and/or periodontally compromised require alteration in the design of the prosthesis.

D. If the remaining dentally sound teeth have been periodontally compromised, two implants and a bridge connected telescopically to the abutments should be employed so that the restoration might still be salvaged should a natural tooth be lost. If the teeth are not periodontally involved, two implants and a self-retained bridge are employed.

E. If the remaining teeth need extensive periodontal or dental treatment and are to oppose the natural teeth, two or three implants connected by interlocks to the natural abutments are used. If a removable prosthesis is present already, one implant connected by an interlock to the natural abutments could be employed as a replacement, reducing the treatment costs.

F. When inadequate quantity or quality of bone is present to permit the use of tissue-integrated prostheses because implants cannot be placed, conventional prostheses are the only alternative. In free end saddle cases, removable prostheses are used. In cases with useful posterior abutments present, a conventional fixed bridge is indicated. If the natural abutments are periodontally and/or dentally badly compromised, a conventional removable prosthesis, with or without extraction of those teeth, is the alternative.

One major advance in the last 2 years when dealing with partially edentulous maxilla is sinus grafting. When there is not enough bone (minimum of 10 mm needed because of the lack of predictability with a 7 mm fixture), a graft is performed to elevate the sinus mucosa.

Various materials have been used but the most predictable should be the use of autogenous bone or autologous bone. In the most posterior portion of the maxilla we use pterygomaxillary fixtures to increase the predictability. In most cases it is necessary to use a long fixture distally inclined to engage the pterygomaxillary phisurae. Very dense bone is formed by the pterygoid process and the vertical part of the palatine bone.

References

Boyne PJ, James RA. Grafting of the maxillary sinus floor with autogenous marrow and bone. J Oral Surg 1980; 6:613.

Damien CJ, Parson JR. Bone graft and bone graft substitutes. A review of current technology and applications. J Appl Biomaterials 1991; 2:187.

Ericsson I, Lekholm U, Branemark P, et al. A clinical evaluation of fixed bridge restoration supported by the combination of teeth and osseointegrated titanium implants. J Clin Periodontol 1986; 13:307.

Lekholm U. Clinical procedures for treatment with osseointegrated dental implants. J Prosthet Dent 1983; 50:1117.

Sullivan D, Krogh P. A solution for the prosthetic problem of the hemidentate arch with tissue integrated prosthesis. Int J Periodontol Restor Dent 1986; 4:66.

Sullivan D. Prosthetic considerations for the utilization of osseointegrated fixtures in the partially edentulous arch. Int J Oral Maxillofac Implants 1986; 1:81.

Tulasne JF. Implant treatment of missing posterior dentition. In The Branemark osseointegrated implant. Quintessence Books; 19:103.

Patient with SOME POSTERIOR EDENTULOUS AREAS IN THE MAXILLA

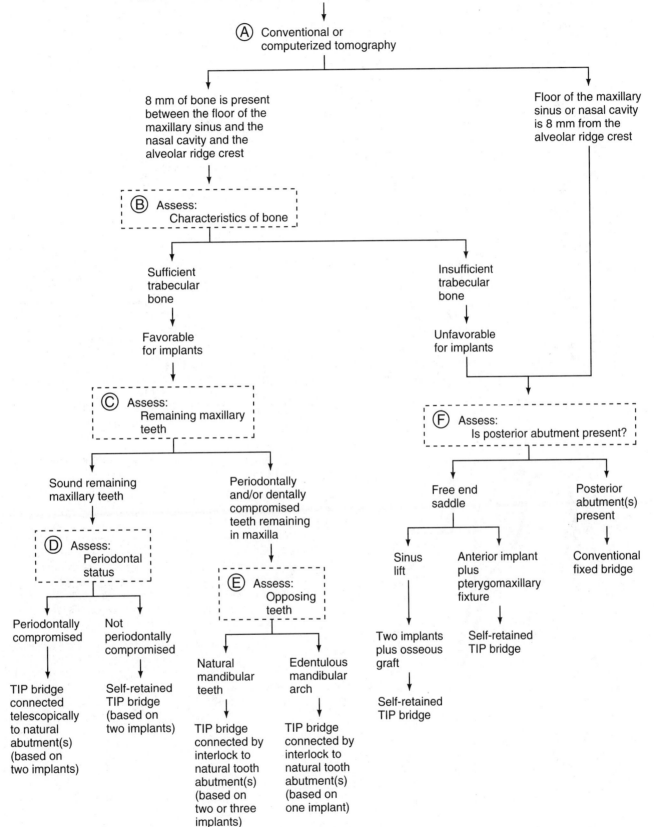

(A) Conventional or computerized tomography

8 mm of bone is present between the floor of the maxillary sinus and the nasal cavity and the alveolar ridge crest

Floor of the maxillary sinus or nasal cavity is 8 mm from the alveolar ridge crest

(B) Assess: Characteristics of bone

Sufficient trabecular bone

Favorable for implants

Insufficient trabecular bone

Unfavorable for implants

(C) Assess: Remaining maxillary teeth

(F) Assess: Is posterior abutment present?

Sound remaining maxillary teeth

Periodontally and/or dentally compromised teeth remaining in maxilla

Free end saddle

Posterior abutment(s) present

(D) Assess: Periodontal status

(E) Assess: Opposing teeth

Sinus lift

Anterior implant plus pterygomaxillary fixture

Conventional fixed bridge

Periodontally compromised

Not periodontally compromised

Natural mandibular teeth

Edentulous mandibular arch

Two implants plus osseous graft

Self-retained TIP bridge

TIP bridge connected telescopically to natural abutment(s) (based on two implants)

Self-retained TIP bridge (based on two implants)

TIP bridge connected by interlock to natural tooth abutment(s) (based on two or three implants)

TIP bridge connected by interlock to natural tooth abutment(s) (based on one implant)

Self-retained TIP bridge

GUIDED BONE AUGMENTATION FOR OSSEOINTEGRATED IMPLANTS

William Becker
Burton E. Becker

The principles of guided tissue regeneration (GTR) used for periodontal regeneration can be used for root form dental implants. The tissue involved in the healing of an extraction socket are flap connective tissue and bone. Membrane barriers may be used to exclude flap connective tissue from collapsing into an extraction socket that has received an immediately placed implant, allowing the necessary cells for bone formation access to the area. The barrier creates a space and protects the clot during the early healing phase, resulting in an environment conducive to bone formation around the portion of the implant that is not fully encompassed by bone (Fig. 1). A specially designed e-otfte membrane (Gore-Tex Augmentation Material [TMJ]) is used for this purpose. The oval-shaped material has an inner portion that is totally occlusive and a peripheral portion that allows for the ingrowth of connective tissue fibrils. Guided bone augmentation (GBA) used with osseointegrated implants has been demonstrated in animal and human clinical studies.

A. Successful use of GBA for implants placed into extraction sockets requires careful case selection. Teeth which have advanced untreatable periodontitis, recurrent endodontic lesions, or fractures that are not exposable by crown lengthening are ideal candidates for extraction followed by immediate implant placement. To obtain maximum implant stability, there should be a minimum of 3 to 5 mm of bone apical to the root tip. Implants placed into thin, edentulous ridges may result in fenestrations. These defects can be treated with GBA.

B. When the site is exposed surgically, the type of defect and site are evaluated and the potential or actual stability of an implant is assessed. If a stable implant cannot be placed, alternative restorative plans should be proposed.

C. Fenestration defects that result from placing the implant close to the facial surface of the implant can be treated with GBA. The implant must be completely stable. If the fenestration exposes only one or two threads, no barrier is necessary. When a large fenestration is present (exposing three or more threads of the implant), a barrier should be placed over the defect for GBA.

D. When an implant has been placed into an extraction socket, an intra-alveolar defect may exist. When implants are placed into extremely narrow sockets (as those present on mandibular anterior teeth) or into extremely wide bone leaving no exposure of the implant in the adjacent socket, no GBA is necessary. Defects less than 3 mm deep that do not expose more than three threads may have a barrier placed. Defects greater than 3 mm deep that expose more than three threads should be considered for GBA.

E. An implant placed into an extraction socket with one or more bony walls missing may be treated with GBA. If two walls cannot be stabilized, it should be removed immediately. Many times one or two bony walls are partially missing, and the implant is stable. This is the ideal defect in which to use GBA.

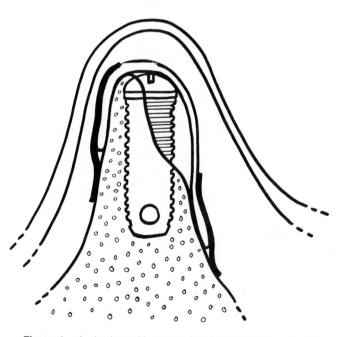

Figure 1. An implant with exposed body knurling covered with a membrane for GBA.

Patient for an OSSEOINTEGRATED IMMEDIATE IMPLANT

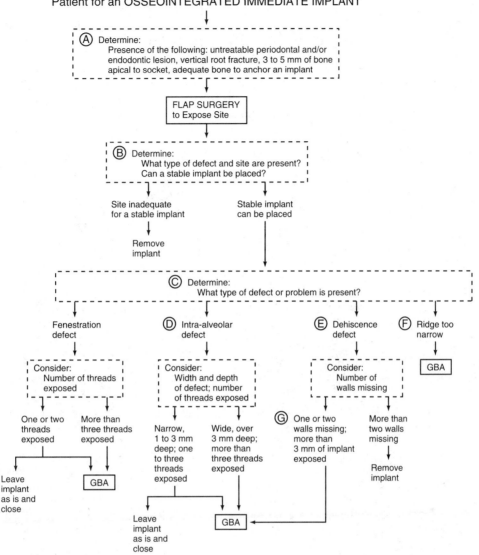

F. When any of the above defects occur in conjunction with a narrow ridge, GBA may be used to attempt to augment the width of the ridge.

G. When barriers are used for implant augmentation, complete flap closure over the barrier should be obtained prior to removal but the barrier occasionally becomes exposed. If a small area becomes exposed prior to 30 days, the area may be cleansed with chlorhexidine swabs. If the barrier has a large exposed area and inflammation is present, it should be removed immediately. The ideal situation exists when the barrier remains completely covered until its removal at 4 to 6 weeks after placement.

References

Becker W, Becker BE, Ochsenbein C, et al. Bone formation at dehisced dental implant sites treated with implant augmentation material: A pilot study in dogs. Int J Periodontol Restor Dent 1989; 9:333.

Becker W, Becker BE, Prichard J, et al. Root isolation for new attachment procedures: A surgical and suturing method: Three cases report. J Periodontol 1987; 58:819.

Dahlin C, Sennerby L, Lekholm U, et al. Generation of new bone around titanium implants using a membrane technique: An experimental study in rabbits. Int J Oral Maxillofac Implants 1989; 4:19.

Gottlow J, Nyman S, Lindhe J. New attachment formation as a result of controlled tissue regeneration. J Clin Periodontol 1984; 11:494.

Lazzara RJ. Immediate implant placement into extraction sites: Surgical and restorative advantages. Int J Periodontol Restor Dent 1989; 9:333.

Nyman S, Lang NP, Buser D, Bragge U. Bone regeneration adjacent to titanium dental implants using guided tissue regeneration: A report of two cases. Int J Oral Maxillofac Implants 1990; 5:9.

PERIMPLANTITIS: ETIOLOGY OF THE AILING, FAILING, OR FAILED DENTAL IMPLANT

Mark Zablotsky
John Kwan

The discipline of implant dentistry has gained clinical acceptance as a result of long-term studies suggesting very high success/survival rates in both partially and completely edentulous applications; however, in a small percentage of cases implant failure and morbidity have been reported. Implant failure due to surgically overheating bone has been minimized with the advent of slow speed, high torque, internally and often externally irrigated drilling systems. After either biointegration or osseointegration the major cause of implant failure is thought to involve a biomechanical (e.g., overload, heavy lateral interferences, lack of a passive prosthesis fit) or infectious (plaque-induced) etiology.

Complications can be eliminated or minimized with adequate treatment planning. Mounted study models with diagnostic waxups or tooth setups are mandatory to evaluate ridge relationships, occlusal schemes, and restorative goals. When these are considered together with adequate radiographs and clinical examination the implant team (restoring dentist, surgeon, and laboratory technician) can adequately plan for the location, number, and trajectory of implants to ensure the most esthetic and functional prosthesis. Often additional implants may be proposed to satisfy the implant team and patient requirements (e.g., fixed versus removable prostheses). The final restoration should be esthetic and adequately engineered (enough implants of sufficient length in sufficient quality and quantity of supporting bone) and allows the patient to perform adequate home care. When evaluating the ailing/failing implant one or more of the above criteria often have not been met.

A. When referring to a dental implant as ailing, failing, or failed, one really is referring to the status of the peri-implant supporting tissues (unless the implant is fractured). The ailing implant displays progressive bone loss and pocketing but no clinical mobility. The failing implant displays similar features to the ailing implant but is refractory to therapy and continues to worsen. This implant is also immobile. The term "ailing" implies a somewhat more favorable prognosis than the term "failing."

B. A failed implant is one that is fractured, has been totally refractory to all methods of treatment, or has clinical mobility and/or circumferential peri-implant radiolucency. These implants must be immediately removed as progressive destruction of surrounding osseous tissues may occur.

C. The etiology of peri-implant disease is often multifactorial. Many times the clinician must search for the potential etiology. Meffert has coined the terms *traditional* versus the *retrograde* pathways when differentiating bacterial versus biomechanical etiologies.

Although a hemidesmosomal attachment of soft tissues to titanium has been reported, it is doubtful that this histologic phenomenon has clinical relevance to titanium implant abutments. The peri-implant seal is thought to originate from a tight adaptation of mucosal tissues around the abutment via an intricate arrangement of circular gingival fibers and a tight junctional epithelium. Because this "attachment" is tenuous at best, it can be extrapolated that a plaque-induced (traditional pathway) peri-implant gingivitis may not truly exist and that plaque-induced inflammation of peri-implant tissues may directly extend to the underlying supporting osseous tissues.

D. The periodontal ligament acts as a "shock absorber" around the natural tooth when excessive occlusal or orthodontic forces are present. In the absence of bacterial plaque, occlusal trauma does not cause a loss of attachment to teeth; however, because implants lack a periodontal ligament, force can be transmitted to the implant/bone interface. If significant enough, microfractures of this interface can occur and allow for an ingress of soft tissues and secondary bacterial infection.

In fixed bridgework that does not fit passively and is cemented on natural teeth, orthodontic movement of abutments occurs due to the presence of the periodontal ligament. In this scenario little if any damage occurs around abutments because of this orthodontic movement. When this same phenomenon occurs on dental implant abutments (either screw-retained or cemented), one of a few complications can result. The restoration may become loose either as a result of cement failure, screws backing out, or fracture. Abutments can loosen or fracture, or the implant body may fracture or have bone loss caused by progressive microfractures at the interface (retrograde pathway); therefore, frameworks must fit precisely. Lateral interferences or excessive off-axis loading can lead to greater stresses on components as well as implant-bone interface and should be minimized. Bruxism can be extremely destructive and should be addressed either by modifying occlusal schemes to eliminate lateral contacts in function or parafunction or the patient should submit to permanent splint/nightguard treatment prior to implant placement. In some instances a removable prosthesis may be used.

When evaluating the ailing/failing implant, clinical signs of peri-implant problems include increased

Patient with INCREASING PROBING DEPTHS AND BONE LOSS AROUND AN IMPLANT

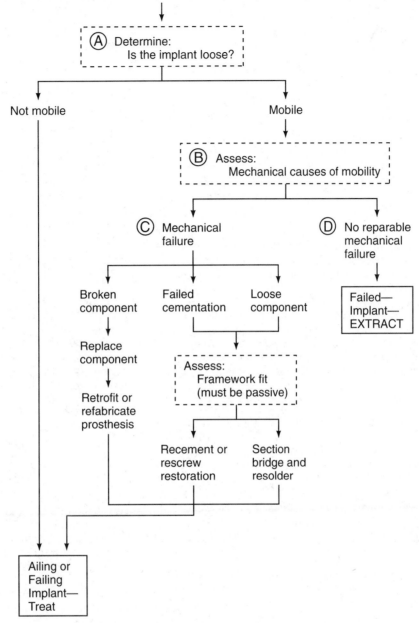

probing depths, bleeding on probing, suppuration, erythema and flaccidity of tissues, and radiographic bone loss. Pain may be present, but usually it is a late symptom. If plaque is absent with minimally inflamed tissues, an occlusal etiology is suspected. Often this can be confirmed via culture and sensitivity testing. If bacteria associated with gingival health are present (e.g., *Streptococcus* spp. or *Actinomyces* spp.), an occlusal component is strongly suggested. If, however, periodontal pathogens (e.g., *P. gingivalis, P. intermedia* etc.) are present, peri-implant infection should be highly suspected; there may also be an occlusal component. Restorations should be inspected for fit. A loose restoration is always a bad sign. Each component must be evaluated and removed until the loose or failed component is found. If the implant is loose, it is a failure and should be immediately

removed. It will never reintegrate and be functional. Replacement implants can be placed either at the time of or within 6 months of implant removal, as various regenerative techniques may be contemplated to maintain alveolar height and width.

References

Meffert R, Block M, Kent J. What is osseointegration? Int J Periodontol Restor Dent 1987; 11(2):88.

Newman M, Fleming T. Periodontal considerations of implants and implant associated microbiota. J Dent Educ 1988; 52(12):737.

Rosenberg E, Torosian J, Slots J. Microbial differences in 2 distinct types of failures of osseointegrated implants. Clin Oral Implant Res 1991; 2(3):135.

INITIAL THERAPY FOR THE AILING/FAILING DENTAL IMPLANT

Mark Zablotsky
John Kwan

A differential diagnosis should be made as early as possible in the initial stages of implant therapy as information garnered may be critical in the followup and maintenance of the ailing/failing implant. If an accurate assessment of the etiology has not been established, any interceptive therapy may be compromised.

A. Effective patient-performed plaque control is mandatory, and the patient must accept this responsibility. The therapist should customize a hygiene regimen for each implant patient. The use of conventional oral hygiene aids (e.g., brush, floss) can be augmented with any number of instruments (e.g., superfloss, yarn, plastic-coated proxibrushes, electric toothbrushes). If the patient's oral hygiene is suspect, the addition of a topical application of chemotherapeutics (e.g., chlorhexidine) either by rinsing or applying locally (e.g., via dipping brushes) may be very beneficial. The restorative dentist must ensure that the patient has access to implant abutments circumferentially.

B. Occlusions should be evaluated, and centric/lateral prematurities and interferences should be eliminated via occlusal adjustment. Nightguard/splint therapy should be initiated if parafunctional activity is suspected. Often, if occlusal etiology is suspected, clinicians remove the prosthesis and place healing cuffs on the implants in hopes of getting a positive response by reducing the load. Single implants that are attached to mobile natural teeth may be overloaded because of the compression of the tooth and subsequent relative cantilevering of the prosthesis from the implant. If occlusal etiology is suspected in such a case, more implants should be contemplated and attached to the existing weakened implant to support the cantilevered/periodontally weak teeth. If bacterial etiology is suspected, initial conservative treatment may consist of subgingival irrigation with a blunt-tipped, side-port irrigating needle. Chlorhexidine is probably the irrigant of choice. Local application of tetracycline via monolithic fibers may be an effective adjunct.

C. Culture and sensitivity testing should be done to guide therapy if systemic antibiotics are contemplated. Local debridement of hyperplastic peri-implant tissues should be considered, utilizing hand or, if the implant/abutment is going to be touched, ultrasonic plastic instrumentation.

D. Ideally, the implant abutment should emerge through attached keratinized mucosa, giving the patient an ideal mucosa. This results in an ideal environment for the patient to perform home care as movable alveolar mucosal margins can be irritated and adversely affect oral hygiene. Increased failures of implants and morbidity have been associated with areas that are deficient in attached keratinized gingival tissues. Soft tissue augmentation procedures can be performed prior to implant placement, during integration, at uncovering (Stage 2), or for repair procedures.

E. Re-evaluation of peri-implant tissues should be done 2 to 4 weeks after initial therapy. Probing depths should be reduced with no bleeding on probing or suppuration present. The clinician must decide whether the improvement in clinical indices is a predictable long-term endpoint. One must remember that the success of periodontal therapy depends on the therapist's ability to remove plaque, calculus, and other bacterial products from radicular surfaces. Because root planing of the implant surfaces is not possible or recommended (because of the detrimental effects of conventional curettes or ultrasonics), the titantium abutment or hydroxylapatite-coated or titanium implant surface must be considered to be contaminated with bacteria and their products (e.g., endotoxin). Therefore, the implant and peri-implant tissues would benefit most from surgical intervention.

If the therapist feels that a successful endpoint has been attained, close maintenance with monitoring of clinical, radiographic, and microbiologic parameters is imperative. Prompt recurrence of problems calls into question either the initial diagnosis (incorrect etiology) or the predictability of the more conservative nonsurgical therapy. In this instance the clinician should strive to stabilize/arrest the active disease process (nonsurgically) and then reevaluate to determine a clinical endpoint. Commonly, cases that are refractory to nonsurgical therapy do well after surgical intervention as the contaminated implant surface can be more readily accessed.

References

Gammage D, Bowman A, Meffert R. Clinical management of failing dental implants: Four case reports. J Oral Implant 1989; 15(2):124.

Kwan J. Implant maintenance. J Calif Dent Assoc 1991; 19(12):45.

Kwan J, Zablotsky M. The ailing implant. J Calif Dent Assoc 1991; 19(12):51.

Orton G, Steele D, Wolinsky L. The dental professional's role in monitoring and maintenance of tissue-integrated prostheses. Int J Oral Maxillofac Implants 1989; 4:305.

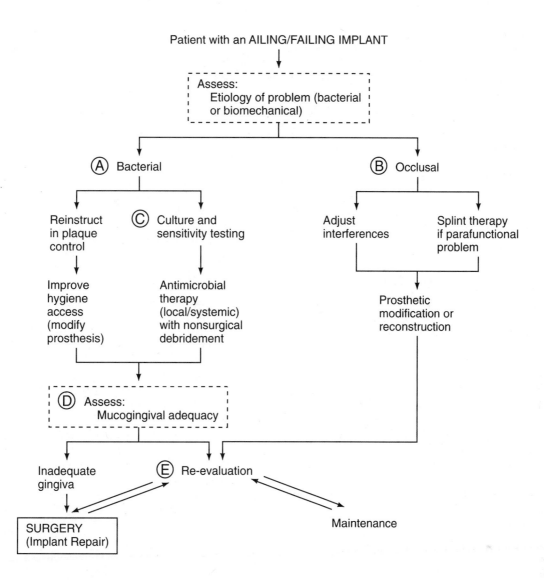

Patient with an AILING/FAILING IMPLANT

Assess:
Etiology of problem (bacterial or biomechanical)

(A) Bacterial

(B) Occlusal

Reinstruct in plaque control

(C) Culture and sensitivity testing

Adjust interferences

Splint therapy if parafunctional problem

Improve hygiene access (modify prosthesis)

Antimicrobial therapy (local/systemic) with nonsurgical debridement

Prosthetic modification or reconstruction

(D) Assess:
Mucogingival adequacy

Inadequate gingiva

(E) Re-evaluation

Maintenance

SURGERY (Implant Repair)

THE SURGICAL MANAGEMENT OF PERIMPLANTITIS: IMPLANT REPAIR

Mark Zablotsky
John Kwan

The surgical repair of the ailing/failing implant is dependent on an accurate diagnosis and effective nonsurgical intervention to stabilize or arrest the progression of the active peri-implant lesion (Figs. 1 to 3).

A. It is important to assess the mucogingival status of peri-implant tissues prior to repair surgery. If only mucogingival defects exist around the ailing/failing implant, osseous repair surgery may not be necessary following soft tissue augmentation around the ailing/failing implant. If indicated, osseous repair surgery is less technically demanding when dealing with keratinized tissues.

B. Modifications of periodontal surgical procedures, either resective or regenerative, have been reported with some success. After making the initial incisions and degranulating the osseous defect (open debridement), one must evaluate the defect prior to selecting the appropriate surgical modality.

C. Peri-implant osseous defects that are predominately horizontal in nature respond most predictably to resective procedures (i.e., definitive osseous surgery) with or without fixture modification.

D. Fixture modification is performed to remove macroscopic or microscopic features that can interfere with subsequent plaque control in the supracrestal aspect of the defect. Fixture modification consists of smoothing with a series of rotary instruments in descending grit (i.e., fine diamond, white stone, rubber points) and using copious irrigation as significant heat can be generated by these instruments. For those with concerns of contaminating implant surfaces or peri-implant tissues with rotary instruments, some have reported a healthy soft tissue response against hydroxylapatite-coated or plasma-sprayed titanium implant surfaces. If the patient's oral hygiene is suspect, fixture modification should be considered for these microscopically rough surfaces.

E. Regenerative procedures (bone grafting with or without guided tissue regeneration [GTR]) have been reported for the repair of the ailing/failing implant. Regenerative procedures are most appropriate when the adjacent osseous crest is close to the rim of the implant (i.e., narrow two- or three-walled moat or dehiscence/fenestration defects). When these procedures are contemplated, fixture modification is not recommended.

F. Detoxification procedures to treat the infected implant surface is recommended prior to regenerative modalities. A 30 second to 1 minute application of a supersaturated solution of citric acid (pH 1) burnished with a cotton pledget appears to be very beneficial in detoxifying the infected hydroxylapatite-coated implant surface. However, if the coating appears pitted and altered, it should be removed either with ultrasonic or air/powder abrasives. A short application of an air/powder abrasive detoxifies the titanium implant surface. Extreme caution is recommended if the defect to be treated with the air/powder abrasive is a narrow intrabony defect, because pressurized air may enter the marrow spaces and create a risk of embolism.

Patient with an AILING/FAILING IMPLANT FOR WHICH SURGERY IS INDICATED

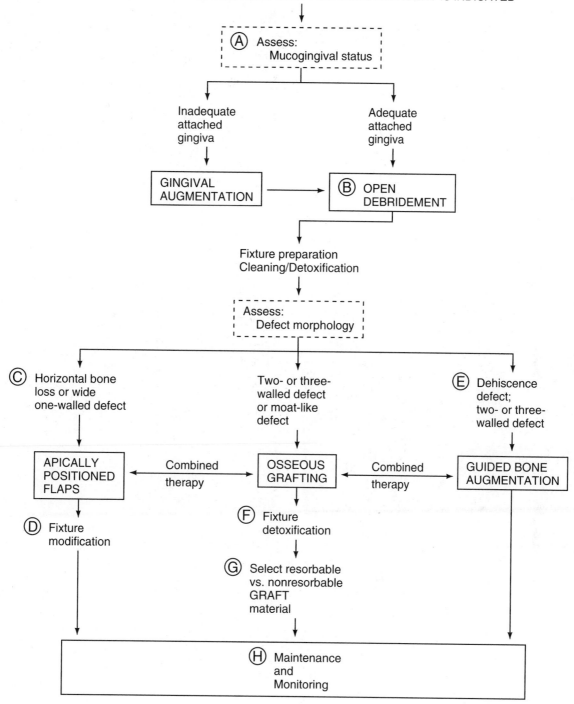

G. Choice of bone grafting materials should be based on the clinician's level of certainty that the site to be grafted is free of bacterial contaminants. If the clinician is certain that the defect is not contaminated, resorbable materials (i.e., autogenous bone, DFDBA, or resorbable hydroxylapatite, or GTR materials alone) may be considered. If the surface of the implant is suspect, nonresorbable materials (i.e., dense nonresorbable hydroxylapatite) should be considered. Nonresorbable bone grafting materials should be used to obturate apical vents and basket holes, as osseous regeneration probably cannot occur in these anatomically contaminated environments.

Combined therapies should be contemplated whenever defect combinations include horizontal bone loss and dehiscence or intrabony defects. Postoperative care is much like that for periodontal surgical procedures, with close follow-up and re-evaluation prior to placement of the patient on a supportive maintenance schedule.

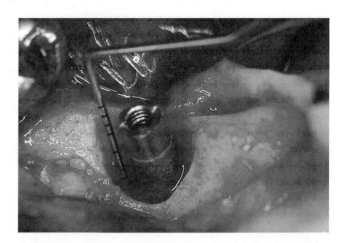

Figure 2. The defect surgically exposed prior to GoreTex membrane placement.

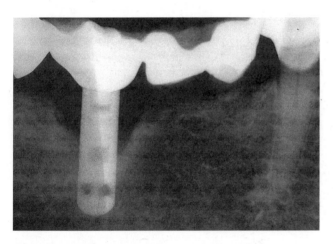

Figure 1. Preoperative radiograph of an "ailing" implant prior to guided bone augmentation repair.

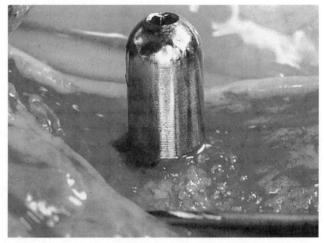

Figure 3. Six months following guided bone augmentation, the defect is filled with hard tissue.

H. The goals of peri-implant surgical and nonsurgical therapies are to re-establish a healthy perimucosal seal and to regenerate a soft or hard tissue attachment to the implant/abutment. This requires a definitive diagnosis, comprehensive therapy, and effective maintenance. At this time no prospective or retrospective studies exist that deal with short- or long-term results attained through implant repair procedures; therefore, close follow-up for recurrence of disease is warranted. Although the goals of therapy are clear, the clinician must be willing to accept and recognize failure when it occurs. The dental implant that is refractory to all treatment attempts is a failure and should be removed as soon as this diagnosis is made.

References

Lozada J, James R, et al. Surgical repair of peri-implant defects. J Oral Implant 1990; 16(1):42.

Meffert R. How to treat ailing and failing implants. Implant Dent 1992; 1:25.

Zablotsky M. The surgical management of osseous defects associated with endosteal hydroxyapatite-coated and titanium dental implants. Dent Clin North Am 1992; 36(1):117.

Zablotsky M, Diedrich D, Meffert R. The ability of various chemotherapeutic agents to detoxify the endotoxin contaminated titanium implant surface. Implant Dent (in press).

Zablotsky M, Diedrich D, Meffert R, Wittrig E. The ability of various chemotherapeutic agents to detoxify the endotoxin infected HA-coated implant surface. Int J Oral Implant 1991; 8(2):45.

TIMING OF RESTORATION FOLLOWING PERIODONTAL SURGERY

Walter B. Hall

The timing of restoration following periodontal surgery depends on the types and objectives of the surgical procedures employed and the use of such presurgical treatment as temporary (up to 6 months) or provisional (up to 2 years) splinting. The type of restoration to be placed and the degree of success of the surgery in meeting its objectives at the time of evaluation also influence timing of postsurgical restoration. New attachment procedures (e.g., guided tissue regeneration, bone fill procedures, and pure mucogingival procedures for root coverage) usually require a longer time (6 months or more) before reevaluation for restoration can be done than do pocket elimination procedures, for which a month may be sufficient. Splinting allows for a longer period in which to evaluate the success of surgical procedures. Restorations that are placed supragingivally do not require as long a wait as those that are placed at the gingival margin or subgingivally.

A. If pure mucogingival surgery is the only surgery planned, the timing of restoration depends only on the goals of the surgical procedure employed. If grafting is done only to increase the band of attached gingiva (i.e., root coverage is not attempted), a wait of only 2 to 4 weeks is adequate before evaluating for restoration. If root coverage is a goal, an evaluation after 6 months or more is necessary to determine whether new attachment (clinically) has been attained.

B. If mucogingival-osseous surgery alone or combined with pure mucogingival surgery is done, reevaluation depends on whether the involved teeth are splinted or not and the objectives of the type of surgery employed.

C. If the involved teeth are temporarily or provisionally splinted, the timing of restoration depends on the type of surgery employed. If guided tissue regeneration (see p 64) or a gingival or connective tissue graft for root coverage is employed, reevaluation before restoration should be done 6 months or more after surgery. If no new attachment surgical procedures are used, the timing of restoration depends on the severity of the involvement of key teeth. If significantly compromised critical teeth are present, reevaluation prior to restoration should be done 6 months or more after surgery; if no new attachment is attempted, a 1 month wait should be sufficient prior to reevaluation for restoration.

D. If the teeth are not splinted but a new attachment procedure is used, the same guidelines as in C pertain. However, if the teeth are not splinted and pocket elimination or modified Widman flap surgery is employed, reevaluation prior to restoration may be performed as soon as 1 month following surgery.

References

Carranza FA. Clinical periodontology. 7th ed. Philadelphia: WB Saunders, 1990:915.

Hall WB. Periodontal preparation of the mouth for restoration. Dent Clin North Am 1980; 25:195.

McFall WT. The laterally repositioned flap—Criteria for success. Periodontics 1968; 5:89.

Nyman S, Lindhe J. A longitudinal study of combined periodontal and prosthetic treatment of patients and advanced periodontal disease. J Periodontol 1979; 50:163.

Schluger S, Yuodelis R, Page RC, Johnson RH. Periodontal diseases. 2nd ed. Philadelphia: Lea & Febiger, 1990: 612, 642, 666.

Seibert JS, Cohen DW. Periodontal considerations in preparation for fixed and removable prosthodontics. Dent Clin North Am 1987; 31:529.

Patient with a COMPLEX DENTAL PROBLEM WHO HAS HAD PERIODONTAL SURGERY

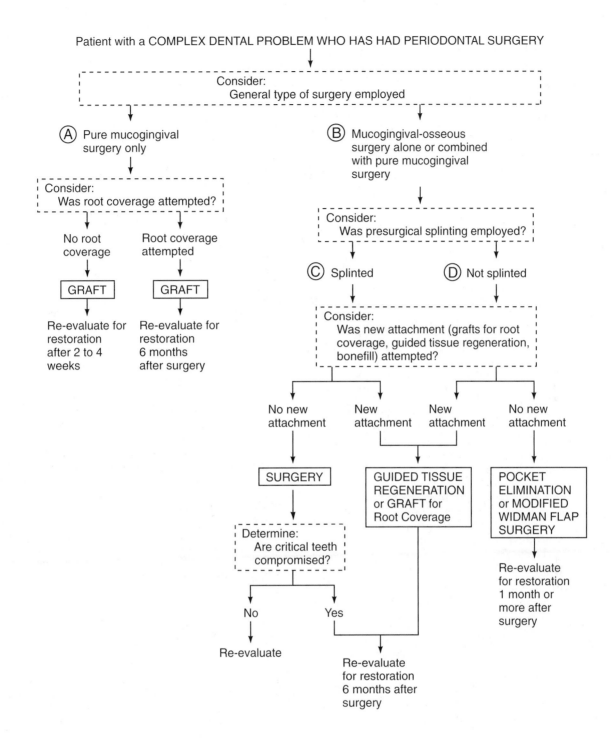

BEHAVIORAL APPROACH TO RECALL VISITS

Walter B. Hall

The timing of recall visits for periodontal patients can be planned in several ways. Some dentists, citing long-term studies of periodontal treatment based on a uniform recall interval, recall all patients at 3 month intervals. They believe that they can predict success rates of various forms of treatment more accurately on this basis; however, the problem with this approach is the patient's response. For years many dentists recalled patients twice a year because studies indicated that between visits caries would not develop so rapidly as to endanger many teeth. In "behavioral" terms, however, many patients "learned" that they had to return to the dentist every 6 months whether they needed it or not (i.e., whether they had made a good effort at oral hygiene or not). Patients understood this message long before dentists did, and oral hygiene and the incidence of caries improved little during that era. An approach that uses the long-term study concepts in a more behaviorally sound way is to "reward" patients depending on the adequacy of their home care efforts between visits; if a patient is doing well (based on assessments of plaque, inflammation, and pocket depth), the time before the next recall is extended, offering a direct reward for individual efforts and reinforcing desirable behavior. With a large group of patients the average recall time is likely to be 3 months; however, no individual patient is likely to be recalled regularly at 3 month intervals.

The greatest advantage of the behavioral approach to recall visit timing is that patients are given an immediate reinforcing "reward" for good or poor effort. The patients can see either that their efforts have paid off or that lack of effort has brought an appropriate "reward." In the fixed interval (every 3 months) approach, only praise or scolding are rewards available to the dentist. The more tangible rewards of less cost (in time, money, and discomfort) is much more likely to prove successful. Additionally, the dentist can demonstrate how the treatment was altered in response to patient behavior between visits and patients must take responsibility for their progress and its costs.

A. When an individual patient's first recall visit is to be scheduled, information on which to base the recall interval is not clearly defined. The patient may have remaining areas of compromise, such as individual teeth for which definitive treatment was impossible (because these teeth already had lost too much attachment) or for which selection of a less definitive treatment was made for financial reasons. Some patients are compromised by the status of their health. Others may be compromised by less than ideal restorative work or tooth alignment. If the patient has areas of compromise, they should be annotated and the recall interval decreased. If a compromised patient has shown little motivation to develop home care skills, the first recall visit should be set at 1 to 2 months; alternatively, if good oral hygiene skill development and motivation are manifested, the first recall can be set at 2 to 3 months. If the patient has no areas of compromise, evidence of oral hygiene skill and motivation can be used to set the first recall interval. If the patient's efforts have been minimally successful, a first recall visit might be set at 2 to 3 months; with greater success the interval could be increased to 3 months or more.

B. Further recall visits are easier to schedule in a behaviorally successful manner. At each recall visit, evaluate plaque control, gingival inflammation status, and pocket depths and use this measure of the patient's "success" to determine the next recall interval. Patient behavior over the years is rarely consistent. Many factors in patients' lives influence their efforts at oral hygiene. Periods of stress or illness affect their ability to deal with plaque. If plaque control has been inadequate, shorten the recall interval. If much inflammation is present and/or pocket depths are increasing, shorten the intervals even more. If the patient's efforts do not improve, alternative approaches (even extraction of poor risk teeth that can endanger adjacent abutments) may be necessary. If efforts improve after several recall visits, an increase in the time between recalls is an appropriate reward. Maintain the current recall interval for a patient whose efforts are fair or adequate. Reward a patient whose efforts have given excellent results by increasing the time between recalls.

References

Chace R. The maintenance phase of periodontal therapy. J Periodontol 1951; 22:23.

Lindhe J. Textbook of clinical periodontology. 2nd ed. Copenhagen: Munksgaard, 1989:615, 626.

Parr RW. Periodontal maintenance therapy. Berkeley: Praxis Publishing, 1974:1.

Ramfjord SP, Knowles JW, Nissle RR, et al. Longitudinal study of periodontal therapy. J Periodontol 1973; 44:66.

Ramfjord SP, Morrison EC, Burgett FG, et al. Oral hygiene and maintenance of periodontal support. J Periodontal 1982; 53:26.

Schluger S, Yuodelis R, Page RC, Johnson RH. Periodontal diseases. 2nd ed. Philadelphia: Lea & Febiger, 1990:732.

Patient with CURRENT PERIODONTAL TREATMENT COMPLETED

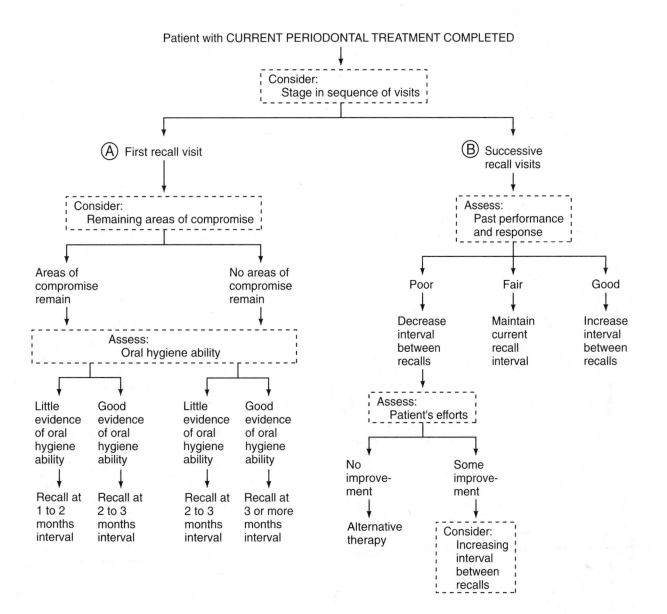

TREATMENT PLANNING FOR THE HUMAN IMMUNODEFICIENCY VIRUS (HIV) POSITIVE PATIENT

Gene A. Gowdey
Walter B. Hall

The increasing life expectancy of human immunodeficiency virus (HIV) positive patients has forced the dentist to reconsider the objectives of dental care for infected persons. Early in the acquired immunodeficiency syndrome (AIDS) era the short life expectancy of infected individuals dictated a treatment plan based on establishing and maintaining patient comfort with as reasonable function as could be attained with as little expense as possible. Now that HIV positive persons may live for many years, the earlier approach must be rethought. As further progress in maintaining life and quality of life is made, treatment planning for growing numbers of HIV positive patients with increasing life expectancies has become an evolutionary process. As understanding and trust progress, the patient and the dentist can deal openly and nonjudgmentally, in the best Hippocratic tradition, to achieve the best dental status possible consistent with the informed wishes and within the means of the patient. Such a treatment planning process can occur only when the dentist knows that the patient is HIV positive.

A. Before a logical treatment plan can be devised, the severity of the patient's systemic problems must be assessed and a current prognosis projected. The patient's blood assay must be analyzed to assess the status of the current health. For example, occasionally, conditions such as thrombocytopenia (a severely depressed platelet count) are seen; thrombocytopenia can lead to prolonged bleeding time or other clotting disorders. In this instance consult with the patient's physician to insure that platelet count is adequate to tolerate a surgical procedure. HIV positive patients often present with abnormal blood assay results that require careful analysis prior to dental or surgical procedures. A dentist wishing to treat HIV positive patients should be thoroughly familiar with normal blood counts and be able to interpret a blood assay; however, all treatment decisions should be made in consultation with the patient's primary care physician.

When treatment planning for the HIV positive patient, a wide spectrum of disease expression can exist (Fig. 1A to F).

B. If the patient is declining significantly such that his life expectancy is short, the severity of his periodontal problems must be assessed or reassessed. Restoring and maintaining comfort through use of chlorhexidine or metronidazole becomes the primary goal. Correction of restorative problems that are symptomatic or compromise nutritional needs is very important too. Major reconstructive plans, however, are not indicated. Palliative treatment becomes the goal.

C. If medical data indicate that the patient is stable, estimates of his long-term prognosis guide dental treatment planning. If in the opinion of the physician, the prognosis still appears guarded, treatment goals must be adjusted to life expectancy prognostications. If the prognosis appears good, where several years of life can be anticipated, however, patient goals and financial considerations become paramount. Many patients receive prophylactic medications that prevent opportunistic infections from shortening their life span. Because of these recent advances, patients are living much longer than previously observed. While developing a treatment plan for HIV-positive patients, bear in mind the possibility of rapid deterioration of the patient's health.

D. If the prognosis is guarded, the patient should be counseled to make his decisions weighing costs and relative benefits to be expected from comprehensive treatment. He may elect to have only palliative treatment if he is pessimistic or puts a low value on dental treatment. If finances are a problem and government assistance is not available, he may have to temper his dental aspirations with fiscal realities. If finances are no problem, only his aspirations need curtail meeting his dental needs.

Many dental infections are merely expressions of opportunistic infections that the patient is experiencing. These oral opportunistic infections (e.g., HIV periodontitis) have a debilitating effect on the patient's overall health. Even chronic periodontitis can drain the patient's immune system and have a deleterious effect on the patient's overall health.

E. For the patient with a good long-term prognosis, dental needs should be presented to him in the same way as presented to any noninfected patient. For example, in the patient with partially erupted third molars, extraction should be considered when the patient's T cell count indicates that healing will occur uneventfully. To wait until a fall in T cell count permits development of severe pericoronitis (Fig. 1, A) would be unwise. Treatment of a smoldering infection that can become acute when immune competency falls is justifiable. The options must be weighed by the dentist and patient intelligently and compassionately. Financial factors may complicate these decisions. Where aid is available, it should be used to satisfy the patient's best interests. When it is not, the dentist must examine his conscience and professional obligations in deciding how to best facilitate necessary care. Some procedures, such as guided tissue regeneration or

Patient with a COMPLEX DENTAL PROBLEM WHO IS HIV POSITIVE

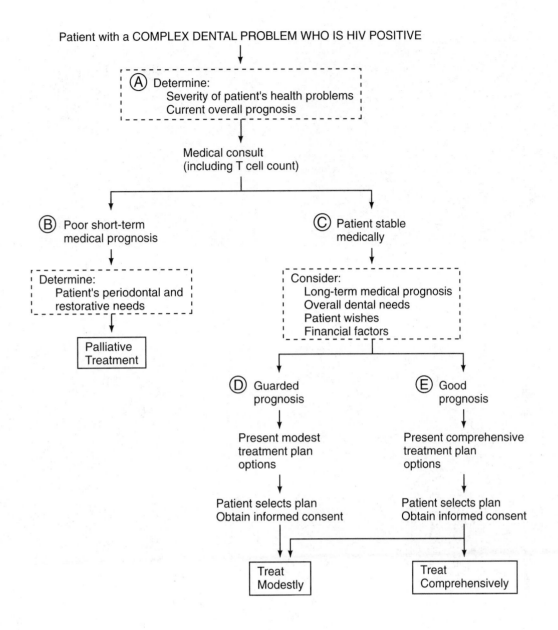

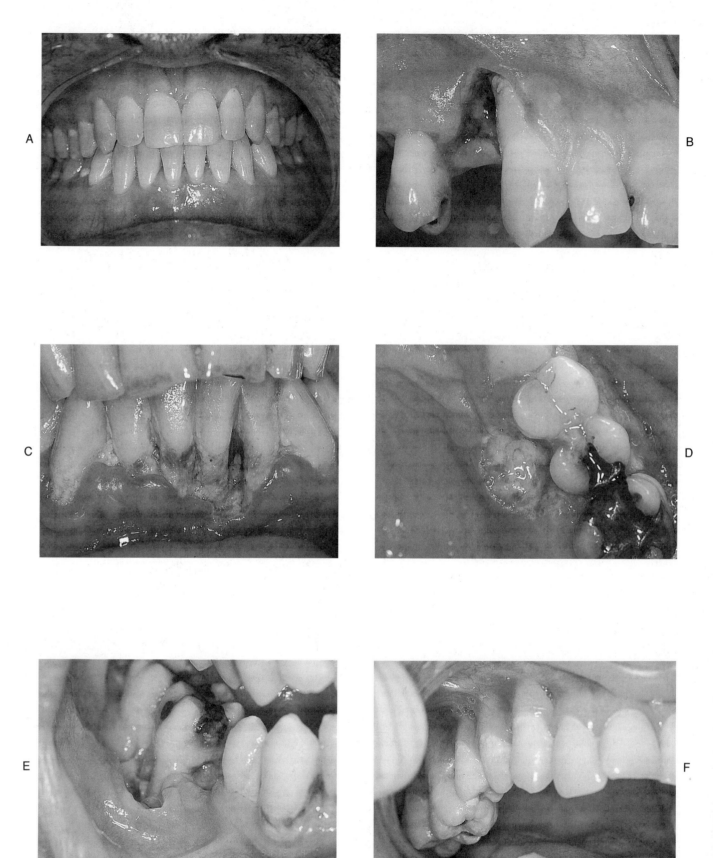

Figure 1. **A,** Perfect health. **B,** HIV periodontitis. **C,** HIV periodontitis with gingival necrosis. **D,** Necrotizing stomatitis. **E,** HIV periodontitis with alveolar bone necrosis. **F,** Vanishing bone phenomenon (total alveolar process disintegration within 8 months). Note the extreme variance from perfect health to advanced debilitation. (Courtesy Dr. Gene Gowdey, San Francisco.)

implant placement, may seem unwise. The risk-to-value ratio of proceeding with such therapy must be explained to the patient in detail and must be reevaluated as knowledge and technique advance so that HIV positive patients with increased life expectancy can receive the best and most appropriate care. Palliative care, such as that which developed in an era when life expectancy was limited, no longer is necessarily the best or only dental care available for HIV positive patients.

References

Greenspan D, Greenspan JS, Pindborg JJ, Schiodt M. AIDS and the mouth. Copenhagen: Munksgaard, 1990.

Pindborg JJ. Classification of oral lesions associated with HIV infection. Oral Surg 1989; 67:292.

Silverman S. Color atlas of oral manifestations of AIDS. Toronto: Decker, 1989.

Silverman S Jr, Migliorati CA, Lozada-Nur F, et al. Oral findings in people with or at high risk for AIDS: A study of 375 homosexual males. J Am Dent Assoc 1986; 112:187.

Winkler JR, Grassi M, Murray PA. Clinical description and etiology of HIV-associated periodontal diseases. In: Robertson PB, Greenspan JS, eds. Perspectives on oral manifestations of AIDS. Diagnosis and management of HIV-associated infections. Littleton, NJ: PSG Publishing, 1988:49.

Winkler JR, Robertson PB. Periodontal disease associated with HIV infection. Oral Surg Oral Med Oral Pathol 1992; 73:145.

ENDODONTICS

Alan H. Gluskin and William W. Y. Goon,
Editors

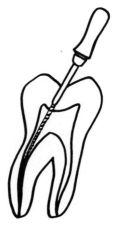

SEQUENCE OF TREATMENT FOR THE PATIENT IN PAIN

Alan H. Gluskin

For many new patients to a dental practice or for patients seeking treatment after many years of neglecting dental care, often the overriding reason for a visit to the dentist is oral pain or toothache.

Whether the etiology of a patient's pain is periodontal, endodontic, or of another origin, the acute emergency treatment is the first therapy the patient receives from the dentist. The treatment plan for comprehensive dental care usually follows.

A. In making a diagnosis of tooth pain, the dentist evaluates the patient's history, reviewing both the medical and dental records. The medical record should suggest any predisposing factors that might contribute to nonodontogenic pain in the head and neck area. Sinus disease, vascular pain syndrome such as migraine, circulatory insufficiencies, trigeminal neuralgia, psychogenic pain, myofascial pain dysfunction, or temporomandibular joint dysfunction all cause radiating pain to the jaws and teeth. In making a differential diagnosis of toothache, the practitioner must understand that nonodontogenic etiologies may coexist with confirmed endodontic and periodontal pathology. This probability must be considered along with any possible odontogenic cause of pain in the patient.

B. In developing a strategy for restoring the patient to optimal oral health, the practitioner must first deal with the patient's acute circumstances and emergency therapy. This may include oral surgery for the extraction of unrestorable or nonsalvageable teeth and initiation of endodontics for acute pulpal and periapical inflammation.

C. For deep lesions, which may compromise pulp vitality, caries control should be a priority equal to an emergency if, early on, it is felt that the tooth can contribute to the overall treatment goals.

D. If pulps are exposed or degenerating, then pulpotomy and or pulpectomy techniques should be used with intermediate restorative materials to bridge the time gap between these procedures and the definitive therapy of endodontics. Unexposed caries control of vital teeth requires pulpal sedation and intermediate restorative materials if the therapy is provided before the treatment plan is finalized.

E. Subsequent to these acute circumstances, an evaluation must be made regarding the periodontal attachment and bony support of teeth. Because periodontal health is the key element in tooth retention and the overall prognosis for teeth, periodontal assessment should be of primary importance in the early stages of the treatment plan.

Once hopeless teeth are identified, those with a better prognosis can be evaluated for worth in the final treatment plan. On occasion, temporary splinting may be required to evaluate salvageability of some mobile teeth while periodontal procedures to manage soft tissue disease is initiated and evaluated. Most complex and varied treatment plans require periodontal therapy as an integral part of the treatment regimen.

A period of time should pass after the emergency therapy is rendered during which the patient is monitored for healing. Then the prognosis for individual abutments in the comprehensive treatment plan can be ascertained.

In summary, endodontic therapy is an integral part of comprehensive patient care. Emergency treatment is initiated early to eliminate acute pulpal and periapical symptoms. Once diagnosis and emergency therapy are accomplished, the teeth can be restored with intermediate materials in order to evaluate healing and develop a treatment plan for comprehensive patient care.

References

Cohen S, Burns R. Pathways of the pulp. 5th ed. St Louis: Mosby–Year Book, 1991:48.

Walton RE, Torabinejad M. Principles and practice of endodontics. Philadelphia: WB Saunders, 1989:69.

Weine FS. Endodontic therapy. 4th Ed. St Louis: CV Mosby, 1989:68.

Patient with a COMPLEX DENTAL PROBLEM WHO IS SYMPTOMATIC OR IN ACUTE PAIN

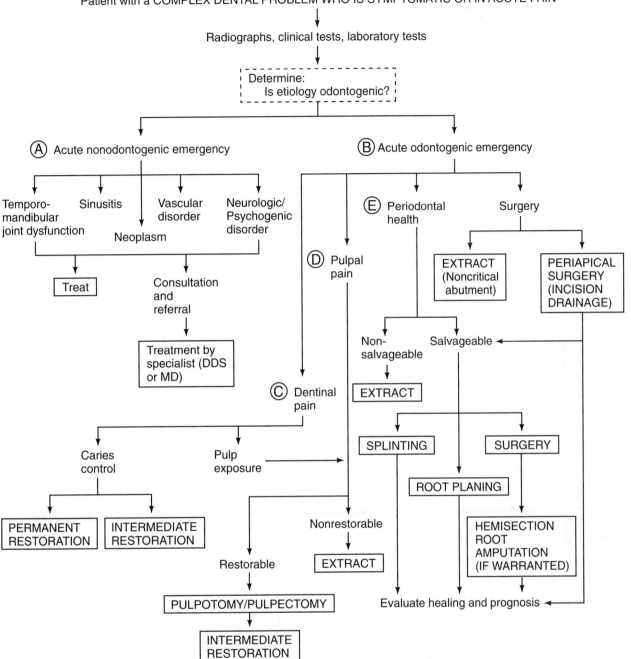

SEQUENCE OF TREATMENT FOR THE ASYMPTOMATIC PATIENT

Alan H. Gluskin

The asymptomatic patient who requires comprehensive dental care to restore oral health may require endodontic procedures in the course of his treatment.

Endodontic therapy is indicated for three main reasons: (1) The asymptomatic tooth with a failing or inadequate root canal filling. (2) Testing or radiographs may disclose an asymptomatic or mildly symptomatic tooth with pulpal or periapical pathology. (3) Endodontics in conjunction with periodontal or restorative procedures may be required on teeth to restore and rehabilitate oral function.

A. Proper timing of comprehensive patient care is critical for proper treatment planning. A priority in comprehensive care is a thorough medical history and evaluation. A patient's physical condition and medications can influence endodontic treatment and ability to heal. As a consequence, a medical history is imperative before any treatment, emergency or otherwise, is initiated.

Comprehensive care is the expected *standard of care* for the patient of record. The scope of care includes evaluation of the medical and dental history as described and a thorough head and neck examination, including soft and hard oral structures.

B. Diagnostic aids (e.g., radiographs, pulp tests, periodontal probing, fiberoptics, percussion and palpation, and additional clinical and laboratory tests) should enable the dentist to diagnose the patient's hard and soft tissue oral problems and develop a problem list. Prioritizing a problem list for the specific task of determining the sequence of treatment is a fundamental principle in comprehensive care. The problem list should also have an underlying organizational efficiency so that more than one procedure in a quadrant can be attempted if this is acceptable to both the dentist and patient.

C. In finalizing the treatment plan the dentist should determine a specific treatment need for each tooth and surrounding area. He must also decide what specialty services might be required. Surgical procedures, such as extractions and ridge alterations, have first priority. Then any mobile and weakened teeth can be splinted prior to periodontal and/or endodontic therapy.

Usually, periodontal therapy such as scaling, root planing and surgery precede final endodontic procedures; however, performing endodontics prior to specific procedures, such as a proposed hemisection or root amputation, offers a much more reliable prognosis. With endodontics completed, the variables in surgical procedures are much more controllable. This is always true for periapical surgery.

Finally, restorative and prosthetic procedures can be initiated when the patient is free from active pathology in the teeth and supporting structures. A short period of time may be required before final restoration in order to clinically and radiographically evaluate periodontal and endodontic healing.

The patient must be maintained in a healthy state by follow-up care at regular intervals, including oral prophylaxis, radiographic recall, and clinical evaluation to monitor continuing health.

In summary, endodontic therapy is an integral part of comprehensive patient care. It must be done early, before restorative work, to evaluate healing and the prognosis of each tooth. It should be integrated in the treatment plan with periodontal therapy as one condition can affect the prognosis of the other.

References

Cohen S, Burns R. Pathways of the pulp. 5th ed. St Louis: Mosby—Year Book, 1991:48.

Walton RE, Torabinejad M. Principles and practice of endodontics. Philadelphia: WB Saunders, 1989:69.

Weine FS. Endodontic therapy. 4th Ed. St Louis: CV Mosby, 1989:68.

Patient with a COMPLEX DENTAL PROBLEM WHO IS ASYMPTOMATIC

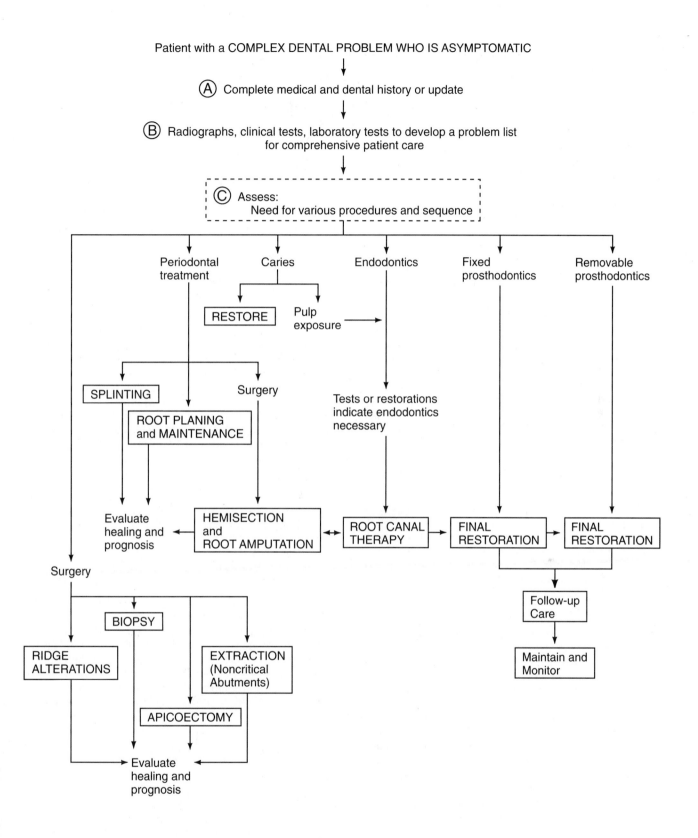

REFERRAL TO AN ENDODONTIST

Alan H. Gluskin

The decision to refer a patient to an endodontist for therapy is made by the general dentist and is an integral part of the delivery of professional care. The thought process in making a referral should involve both technical and nontechnical considerations. Technical factors relate to the difficulty in accomplishing endodontic treatment relative to the biomechanical aspects of therapy. The dentist must consider his own level of training and experience, as well as his diagnostic judgment, before proceeding with any endodontic procedure. Nontechnical factors involve the patient's desires and include management difficulties and health complications that might impact on therapy and postoperative repair and healing.

An underlying factor in all decision making is the principle of *standard of care,* defined as the care that a reasonably prudent practitioner would perform under the same or similar circumstances. When endodontic treatment is provided, all practitioners, whether they are general dentists or specialists, are judged by the same criteria and must render care to the same standards, namely that of the endodontist. Hence general dentists should select and treat only those cases for which they have the training and experience and refer all others.

Once the clinician and patient determine that the problem tooth can be saved by endodontic therapy, the practitioner should consider a list of criteria in determining whether referral is indicated. The patient's best interest is always primary.

A wide range exists in the types of cases a dentist might refer. The potential for an adverse reaction or a procedural mishap in endodontics is very high. Severe pain and prolonged suffering can quickly ruin a doctor/patient relationship, which may have taken years to develop.

A. If the patient presents with a dental emergency, immediate attention is required. Such cases include toothache, pulpal exposures, swelling, and trauma. The dentist with a busy schedule may have little or no time to handle this scenario and maintain the standard of care; thus he should elect to refer.

B. The patient presents with a complex case involving one or more of the following difficulties: a toothache for which the cause is difficult to determine; calcified canals or pulp chambers or complex root and canal morphology; teeth that have had prior procedural accidents, such as perforations and/or separated instruments; retreatment cases with silver cones or hard pastes; traumatized teeth with resorption or immature apices; critical abutments or teeth requiring access through crowns; and complex surgical cases. The dentist must decide if his experience and training are adequate to treat the problem. Referral of such cases allows the patient to benefit from the greater experience of the endodontist.

C. Although there are almost no medical contraindications to endodontic therapy, medically compromised patients who have circulatory disease, bleeding disorders, pulmonary or liver disease, diabetes, adrenal insufficiency, pregnancy, allergies, and/or are receiving radiation or chemotherapy for an immunologic impairment (e.g., caused by HIV or cancer) can be treated quickly and efficiently by the endodontist, making interappointment complications less likely.

D. In addition, a general dentist may wish to refer patients who exhibit management problems (those who are mentally compromised by phobias about dentistry or have true psychologic or mental disorders). Fearful patients can become impossible to calm or even anesthetize if they sense that the general dentist is unfamiliar or uncomfortable with an endodontic procedure. Sedation may be indicated in such a patient, with therapy rendered by a specialist. Many of these psychologic conditions can be overcome by the practitioner who shows a compassionate and caring manner and can develop the patient's trust. In this capacity a general dentist may have as much ability as the endodontist; however, to put the patient at ease and remove stress from the dentist, these patients should be referred to specialists to expedite treatment.

In summary, the prudent general dentist should attempt to select cases that will proceed smoothly and routinely and refer those that may present biomechanical or management difficulties.

The wisest time to make a referral of a potentially problematic case is before that case has been started. The dentist-patient relationship can be quite fragile and have litigious consequences if there is a perceived or real lack of diagnostic or clinical expertise on the part of the dentist. Patients have very little to do with decision making in the referral process and must place a great deal of trust in the general dentist and the proposed specialist to provide the highest quality of treatment to correct their problems.

References

Cohen S, Burns R. Pathways of the pulp. 5th ed. St Louis: Mosby–Year Book, 1991:48.

Dietz GC Sr, Dietz GC Jr. The endodontist and the general dentist. Dent Clin North Am, 1992; 36:459.

Walton RE, Torabinejad M. Principles and practice of endodontics. Philadelphia: WB Saunders, 1989:69.

Weine FS. Endodontic therapy. 4th ed. St Louis: CV Mosby, 1989:68.

Patient who NEEDS ENDODONTIC THERAPY

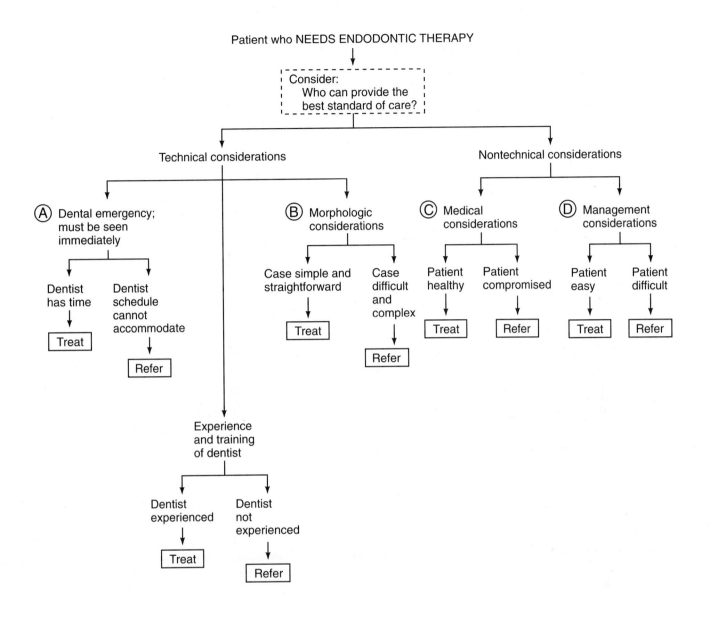

Consider:
Who can provide the
best standard of care?

Technical considerations

Nontechnical considerations

(A) Dental emergency;
must be seen
immediately

Dentist
has time

Treat

Dentist
schedule
cannot
accommodate

Refer

(B) Morphologic
considerations

Case simple and
straightforward

Treat

Case
difficult
and
complex

Refer

(C) Medical
considerations

Patient
healthy

Treat

Patient
compromised

Refer

(D) Management
considerations

Patient
easy

Treat

Patient
difficult

Refer

Experience
and training
of dentist

Dentist
experienced

Treat

Dentist
not
experienced

Refer

PERIODONTAL-ENDODONTIC RAMIFICATIONS OF THE RADICULAR GROOVE: RECOGNITION, DIAGNOSIS, AND PRACTICAL MANAGEMENT

William W. Y. Goon

Progressive localized periodontal disease inevitably develops alongside a radicular groove because of its intimate association with the periodontal sulcus. Maxillary incisors, in particular the lateral incisor, are predisposed to this developmental defect, which begins on or alongside of the cingulum and courses apically onto the root. A myriad of periodontal and endodontic manifestations, ranging from mild to severe, can arise as a result of this defect.

A. A diagnosis of a radicular groove must begin with a thorough intraoral examination of the lingual aspects of all incisor crowns. The periodontal sulcus of incisors with a visually pronounced cingulum should be examined for the presence of localized periodontal disease and carefully probed in its entirety to help disclose any invagination on the tooth or root surface (Fig. 1).

B. Radiographic discernment of parapulpal lines is diagnostic and should alert the astute clinician to search diligently for a grooved defect. The presence of a parapulpal line can easily be confused with an accessory root, an additional root canal, or a vertical root fracture yet often signifies a deeply invaginated defect (Fig. 2).

C. A shallow groove and a short groove have the best long-term prognosis. A parapulpal line is not likely associated with the tooth. Effective management consists of periodontal root planing, gingivectomy to the apical extent of the shallow groove, and plaque control.

D. A moderately long groove or one that is invaginated are often associated with advanced periodontal disease. Periodontal manifestation is influenced by the defect's length and severity. Periodontal management may require a combination of flap elevation, odontoplasty of the groove, filling or sealing the groove with restorative materials or sealants, osteoplasty, guided tissue regeneration, or repositioning the flap. Long-term plaque control is necessary in follow-up care. The success rate is enhanced when the groove is not excessively long and the pulp's vitality is not compromised by root alteration or filling procedures.

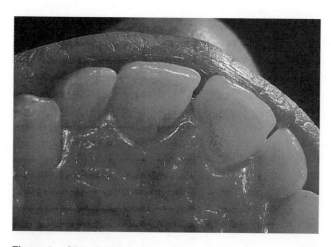

Figure 1. Clinical presentation of the maxillary right central incisor with an invaginated defect which traverses from the cingulum of the crown and courses apically onto the root. The tooth is not fully erupted into the adult occlusion.

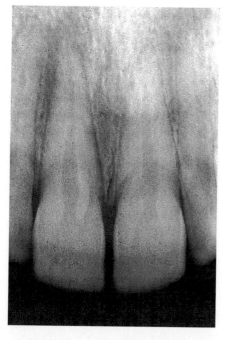

Figure 2. Radiographic evidence of the radicular defect is demonstrated by a parapulpal line coursing mesioapically beyond the cervical level of the crown. Although the tooth is free from decay, the presence of the periapical lesion portrays the adverse endodontic-periodontal implications of the anatomical groove.

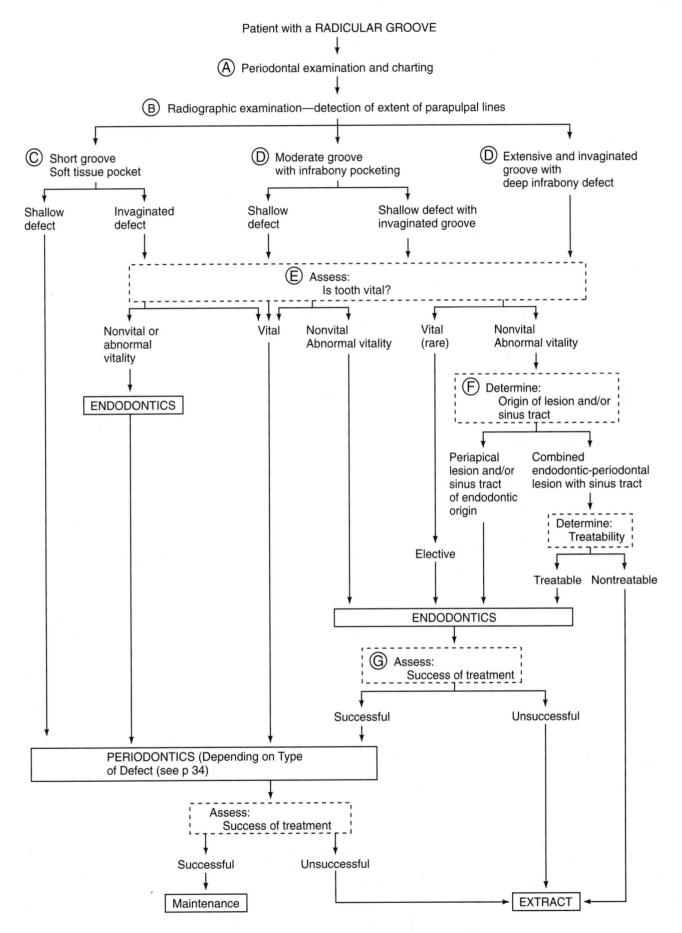

E. An endodontic assessment of the vitality of the pulp is mandatory for any tooth with a deeply invaginated groove or one that radiographically demonstrates a parapulpal line. Some deeply invaginated grooves are defective, permitting direct bacterial entry into the root canal space. This can occur before or concomitantly with the insidious development of a localized periodontal pocket. Similarly, odontoplasty or groove-filling procedures can adversely affect the pulp's vitality, which must be continually monitored. The endodontic assessment of vitality can help to better sequence periodontal management by identifying and electively eliminating the endodontic factor before it becomes firmly established and a liability in the periodontal management.

F. Some invaginated grooves are discovered late and have established endodontic-periodontal disease. Many of these grooves involve most of the root's length. An infrabony pocket is associated with the defect, and a draining sinus tract of endodontic origin is not uncommon. The condition mimics genuine endodontic-periodontal disease, but, unless the radicular groove is detected and diagnosed, treatment will be ineffectual or compromised. Management of a groove with combined endodontic-periodontal disease is determined by the endodontic outcome. Without a favorable response to endodontic therapy, periodontal endeavors cannot be completely effective. A tooth with a radicular groove that is refractory to endodontic and periodontal treatment should be extracted.

G. Occasionally, there is a need to assess a postendodontic failure and the nonresolution of an associated sinus tract and periapical lesion. It is common to find an incisor intact, except for the endodontic access preparation. A radicular groove may have been misdiagnosed as the underlying etiology. The ability to radiographically visualize a parapulpal line, however, is now seriously hampered by the overlapping root canal filling; therefore, an intraoral inspection is mandatory. If a groove is detected, treatment should be terminated and the patient should be advised of the poor prognosis for tooth retention.

References

Everett FG, Kramer GM. The distolingual groove in the maxillary lateral incisor; a periodontal hazard. J Periodontol 1972; 43:352.

Gao Z, Shir J, Wang Y, Gu F, et al: Scanning electron microscopic investigation of maxillary lateral incisors with a radicular lingual groove. Oral Surg 1989; 68:462.

Goon WWY, Carpenter WM, Brace NM, Ahlfeld RJ. Complex facial radicular groove in a maxillary lateral incisor. J Endodon 1991; 17:244.

Lee KW, Lee EC, Poon KY. Palatogingival grooves in maxillary incisor. A possible predisposing factor to localized periodontal disease. Br Dent J 1968; 121:14.

Prichard JS. A textbook of advanced periodontal therapy. Philadelphia: WB Saunders, 1965:14.

Simon JHS, Glick DH, Frank AL. Predictable endodontic and periodontal failures as a result of radicular anomalies. Oral Surg 1971; 31:823.

ENDODONTIC CONSIDERATIONS IN SELECTING OVERDENTURE ABUTMENTS

William W. Y. Goon

Adjunctive endodontic treatment may be required when the comprehensive treatment plan includes a tooth-supported complete denture. The primary beneficiary is the terminal dentition that is severely ravaged by tooth loss and advanced periodontal disease. Teeth in the terminal dentition can be salvaged by removal of the clinical crown, saving the residual root to serve as an abutment supporting the overdenture.

A. Any tooth that is a potential overdenture abutment must undergo an endodontic assessment. The drastic reduction of the coronal tooth structure will unavoidably involve the root canal space.

   An assessment of the patient is also required. The success of the overdenture favors the patient who is truly committed to restoring and maintaining optimum oral health. Patient compliance with the vigorous home care regimen is expected and must include strict oral hygiene of periodontal tissues and daily applications of topical fluoride on exposed natural tooth structure. Regular follow-up visits to review and revise the home maintenance measures and in-office application of silver nitrate in the patient with a high caries index are also necessary. Carelessness in assessing the patient can result in the oversight of a physical impairment, a systemic disease, or potential noncompliance in performing meticulous home care. Perhaps this is the reason for the present neglect and the consideration for denture.

   Also, the dentist must assess his ability to render this type of service and his willingness to provide follow-up support and encouragement to the patient on home maintenance. The dentist who is unable to carry out this professional mandate should get additional training or refer the patient to a practitioner who is capable of overseeing the patient's health and welfare.

B. The terminal status of teeth considered for overdenture abutments requires that the economic burden to the patient be kept to the absolute minimum. The ideal abutment is the single-rooted tooth whose root is structurally sound. The canine tooth is the ideal choice. Its "corner" location in the dental arch and the size and length of the root make it the most strategic tooth to retain. The premolar should be considered when the canine is not available. The incisors are a second choice.

   Superseding the economic consideration are cases in which only a tooth-supported complete denture is the best option for rehabilitating the patient. Success of the overdenture may hinge on salvaging a less desirable tooth for abutment service, perhaps in the presence of a physical impairment or systemic disease. The overriding strategic value of having this abutment warrants a financial commitment to render a successful outcome. Less desirable abutments include the multirooted posterior tooth and a severely compromised root with poor bone support.

C. Unfortunately, the patient requiring an overdenture seldom presents with ideal teeth readily available for abutment service. Often the vestiges of a neglected dentition are all that remain. To devise a functional treatment plan, priority in abutment selection is given first to:

   1. A single-rooted tooth that can sustain the required coronal reduction without needing endodontic treatment. Roots with extensively receded or completely obliterated root canals are viable choices.
   2. A single-rooted tooth that already has a successful endodontic filling is the next logical choice.
   3. Finally, the single-rooted tooth that can be easily treated endodontically can be selected as an overdenture abutment.

D. A single root of a periodontally compromised multirooted posterior tooth may be considered for abutment service following the same priority as for the single-rooted tooth. If indicated, root amputation of the least strategic root(s) can transform the salvaged root into an acceptable abutment. Consideration should be given to the posterior tooth with divergent roots that is amenable to root amputation. This abutment may require associated periodontal procedures to return the tissue to optimum health.

E. The extreme case involves the heroic stabilization of a severely weakened root through an endodontic implant. The root so treated may require additional operative and/or periodontal procedures to retard the progression of periodontal and caries breakdown. An endodontic implant in roots with essentially a questionable prognosis involves the greatest monetary investment and risk of failure.

F. The longevity of an overdenture abutment is significantly increased through a vigorous home care program. Recurrent decay and salivary percolation into the root canal space are the greatest liability to maintaining the integrity of the endodontic seal at the root end. The periodontium must be aggressively maintained in an optimum state of health with meticulous oral hygiene. The susceptibility of exposed root surface of the abutment to caries breakdown can be chemically controlled with daily applications of topical fluoride and fluoride oral rinses. Close supervision and reinforcement of home care techniques are parts of an on-going process that is tailored specifically to each patient.

Patient with a TERMINAL DENTITION REQUIRING OVERDENTURE

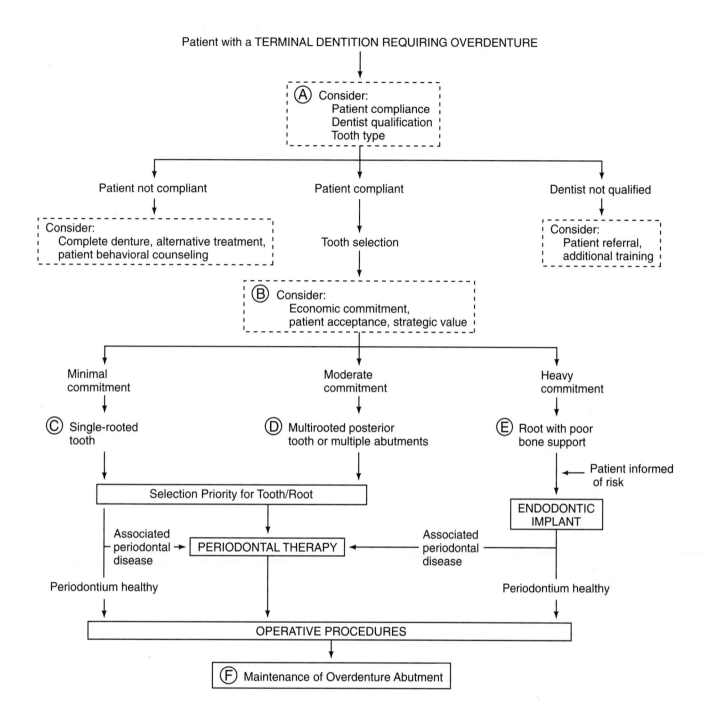

References

DeFranco RL. Overdentures. In: Winkler S, ed. Essentials of complete denture prosthodontics. Philadelphia: WB Saunders, 1979:581.

Grossman LI, Oliet S, Del Rio CE. Endodontic practice. 11th ed. Philadelphia: Lea & Febiger, 1988:346.

Radke RA, Eissmann HF. Postendodontic restoration. In: Cohen S, Burns RC, eds. Pathways of the pulp. 5th ed. St Louis: Mosby, 1991:675.

Trabert KC, Cooney JP, Caputo AA, et al. Preparations for overdentures. In: Ingle JI, Taintor JF, eds. Endodontics. 3rd ed. Philadelphia: Lea & Febiger, 1985:847.

THE ENDODONTICALLY ADEQUATE ABUTMENT TOOTH: A EUROPEAN VIEW

Borja Zabalegui

When a patient has an endodontically involved tooth that is a strategic abutment in a complicated restorative case, the dentist must decide whether the tooth is endodontically treatable or not and whether the successfully treated tooth will be adequate for use in the planned restoration. The endodontic treatment may be surgical or nonsurgical.

A. The involved tooth is first assessed radiographically and clinically. If root canal therapy can be completed successfully or the tooth can be retreated successfully, nonsurgical treatment is preferable (see p 126). If root canal therapy has not or cannot be performed successfully, surgical endodontics (apicoectomy) may be employed to resolve the problem (see p 124).

B. Next, the restorability of the tooth is assessed. If crown lengthening is needed to provide an adequate base for restoration, the dentist must decide whether the tooth can retain adequate support to function as an abutment. If so, proceed with endodontics and crown lengthening in sequence as appropriate (e.g., lengthening before endodontics so a rubber dam can be placed). If not, the tooth should be extracted.

C. If apicoectomy is to be employed, the remaining crown/root ratio must be adequate to function as an abutment. The crown-to-root ratio and the length of span must interrelate such that the abutment will not be traumatized in function. A postcrown is less satisfactory than a nonpost-crown, because post crowned teeth may be more prone to fracture. A cast postretained crown is the least predictable (see p 132). If sufficient support would remain following apicoec-

tomy or apicoectomy and crown lengthening, the appropriate sequencing of endodontics, crown lengthening, and apicoectomy can be developed. If both surgical procedures can be done at once, time and discomfort may be minimized. If the remaining tooth support following one or both of the surgical procedures is inadequate, an alternative restorative plan should be developed. The availability of additional abutments, so that double abutting can be utilized, would enhance the predictability of success as an abutment. If surgery and/or double abutments fail to provide adequate foundations, then the plan may evolve into extracting the tooth or incorporating the tooth in a way that it may still be useful (e.g., an overdenture abutment).

References

Hunter AJ, Feiglin B, Williams JF. Effects of post placement on endodontically treated teeth. J Prosthet Dent 1989; 62:166.

Lord JL, Teel S. The overdenture: Patient selection, use of copings and follow-up evaluation. J Prosthet Dent 1977; 32:41.

Moffa JP, Rossano MR, Doyle MG. Pins—A comparison of their retentive properties. J Am Dent Assoc, 1969; 78:529.

Radke RA, Eissmann HF. Postendodontic restoration. In: Cohen S, Burns RC, eds. Pathways of the pulp. 5th ed. St Louis, Mosby, 1991:640.

Ruddle CJ. Endodontic considerations for periodontal prostheses. CDA J 1989; 41:17.

Patient with an ENDODONTICALLY INVOLVED TOOTH THAT WILL FUNCTION AS AN ABUTMENT

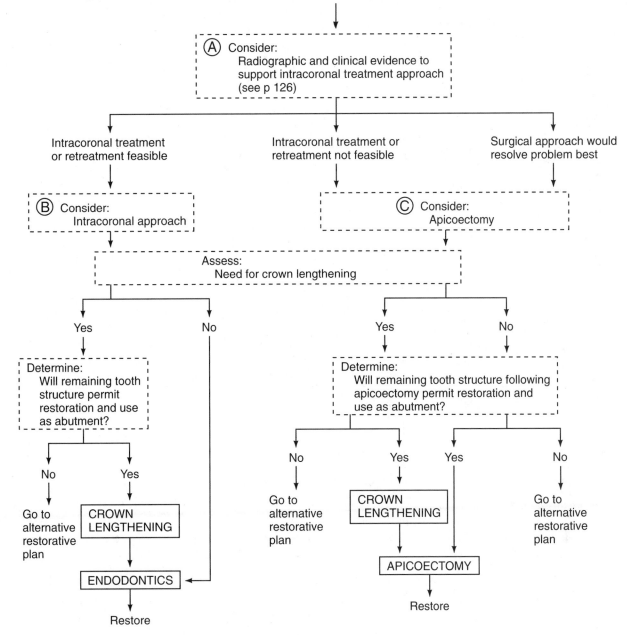

CORONAL MISHAPS ON ENDODONTIC ACCESS: RECOGNITION AND MANAGEMENT

William W. Y. Goon

Iatrogenic defects of the clinical crown can occur when attempting an endodontic access into the tooth. The failure to preplan the best approach to execute and the unwillingness to stop and reassess the alignment of the entry are common factors leading to damage to the crown. Also, full coronal coverage and calcific degenerative closure of the pulp space can handicap even the best attempts at direct access into the chamber of these teeth.

The procedural accident is preventable or can be minimized in the majority of cases. Preplanning is key to avoiding this mishap. The tooth must be thoroughly assessed as to its general anatomy, cervical dimensions, arch, and occlusal alignments. The findings are supplemented with a radiographic assessment of the size, shape, and height of the pulp chamber within the crown. Mental imaging of the radiographic long axis of the submerged root against the clinical crown can give a better sense of root alignment for advantageous positioning of the operative bur.

Three supragingival defects are commonly produced by a misaligned bur. Although the prognosis for tooth retention is favorable, the severity of the defect requires careful consideration in the restoration of the crown.

A. The crown that is gouged has been violated internally. If the root canal system can be located and treated, the crown should be restored with appropriate materials that can withstand the masticatory load for the tooth. An amalgam filling is less likely to flex and can allow the tooth to function without further impairment. The tooth should be monitored for stress fractures of the remaining tooth structure.

B. The crown that is gouged extensively is mutilated internally. Treatment considerations involve the need for full coronal coverage and reinforcement with a post once the endodontic procedure is completed. The tooth should be monitored for horizontal stress fracture of the crown and post.

C. The crown that is perforated, regardless of size, should be temporarily patched to control salivary contamination of the root canal system. The extent of the internal defect (small gouges versus mutilation) governs how the crown is to be restored (see above). The proximity of the defect to the interproximal soft tissue or the gingival sulcus may render the area inaccessible to effective oral hygiene and thus susceptible to caries. Prior to definitive restorative procedures, consideration of crowning lengthening procedures or orthodontic extrusion may facilitate the exposure of the defect for improved oral hygiene or enhance the longevity of the full coronal coverage (see p 134).

References

Bakland LK. Endodontic mishaps: Perforations. Calif Dent Assoc J 1991; 19(4):41.

Frank AL. Resorption, perforations, and fractures. Dent Clin North Am 1974; 18(2):465.

Torabinejad M. Endodontic mishaps: Etiology, prevention, and management. Alpha Omegan 1990; 83:42.

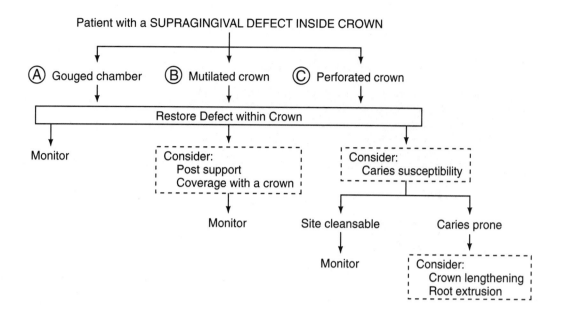

Patient with a SUPRAGINGIVAL DEFECT INSIDE CROWN

(A) Gouged chamber   (B) Mutilated crown   (C) Perforated crown

Restore Defect within Crown

Monitor

Consider:
  Post support
  Coverage with a crown

Monitor

Consider:
  Caries susceptibility

Site cleansable   Caries prone

Monitor

Consider:
  Crown lengthening
  Root extrusion

FURCAL PERFORATION UPON ENDODONTIC MANIPULATION: RECOGNITION, MANAGEMENT, AND PROGNOSIS FOR TOOTH RETENTION

William W. Y. Goon

A perforation into the furcation, also referred to as *cervical canal perforation,* is a significant injury to the periodontal apparatus. A misdirected bur, excessive or misguided postspace preparation, inappropriate widening of the canal orifice or flaring of the coronal canal space, and fruitless searches in a receded pulp chamber for heavily calcified root canal spaces are factors leading to perforations into the furcation. The size and location of the defect are unpredictable and varies according to the particular endodontic procedure attempted. Accessibility to and the sealability of the defect can be troublesome. Inadequate management of the defect is an adverse event and is identified as the second greatest cause of endodontic failure.

A. Upon detection, cursory triage must be initiated to evaluate the impact that the mishap may have on the original treatment plan and the strategic value of the tooth with and without corrective intervention. An extensive defect in a tooth with little strategic value should lead to consideration for extraction. Intact adjacent neighboring teeth should be used instead. A strategic tooth that is important to the overall success of the treatment plan must be evaluated for its long-term prognosis following corrective intervention and the successful completion of the intended endodontic treatment. The prognosis for tooth retention favors the multirooted tooth with a long root trunk. In the tooth with a short root trunk root amputation or hemisection may be a more expeditious and predictable recourse.

B. In considering corrective intervention, the configuration of the perforation determines the accessibility to and the ease and effectiveness of sealing the defect. A small defect or a narrow defect is more amenable to sealing by condensing Cavit, IRM, amalgam, or gutta-percha with sealer cement into the site. A large or broad defect exposes a wide surface wound with little or no retentive features. The placement of sealing materials over the defect must be balanced with sufficient condensing pressures to prevent gross extrusion of material into the furcation and to produce a tight seal of the defect.

C. The tooth that is perforated should be immediately sealed up on or soon after discovery of the mishap.

The objective is to prevent further irritation to and advert deterioration of the exposed and still intact periodontal attachment tissues. Control hemorrhaging by lining the defect with calcium hydroxide, Cavit, Gelfoam, or tricalcium phosphate as a necessary first step to regain direct visualization of the area to make a definitive assessment. The defect should be sealed with amalgam (preferred), Cavit, or gutta-percha and sealer at this time. Ultimately, an effective seal of the defect, rather than the material used, is decisive for a successful repair.

D. The prognosis is favorable for the tooth with a newly discovered defect that is sealed immediately; however, early intervention may not preclude subsequent migration of gingival sulcular epithelium and periodontal pocket formation adjacent to the level of the sealed perforation within 24 months following corrective procedures. This complication is frequently associated with a short root trunk. Surgical curettage and, perhaps, retrograde sealing of the defect or root amputation are the remaining treatment options for salvaging the tooth.

E. The prognosis is less favorable for the perforation that is discovered late and has significant breakdown of osseous supporting tissues. Although circumstances are less desirable, osseous breakdown does not necessarily preclude the salvageability of the tooth, especially one with a long root trunk. The defect should be sealed by filling the osseous cavity with tricalcium phosphate, Gelfoam, or hydroxylapatite to the level of the dental tissue to serve as a matrix for sealing with amalgam. The tooth is closely monitored for osseous regeneration and reformation of the attachment apparatus. Gross extrusion of amalgam into or nonresolution or further deterioration of the osseous tissues warrants consideration of the following treatment options: (1) attempting osseous barrier induction with calcium hydroxide; (2) intentional replantation with direct sealing of the defect; (3) surgical curettage, retrograde seal and, perhaps, a hydroxylapatite graft into the osseous defect; (4) root amputation; and (5) tooth extraction.

PERFORATION OF THE FURCATION ON TREATMENT

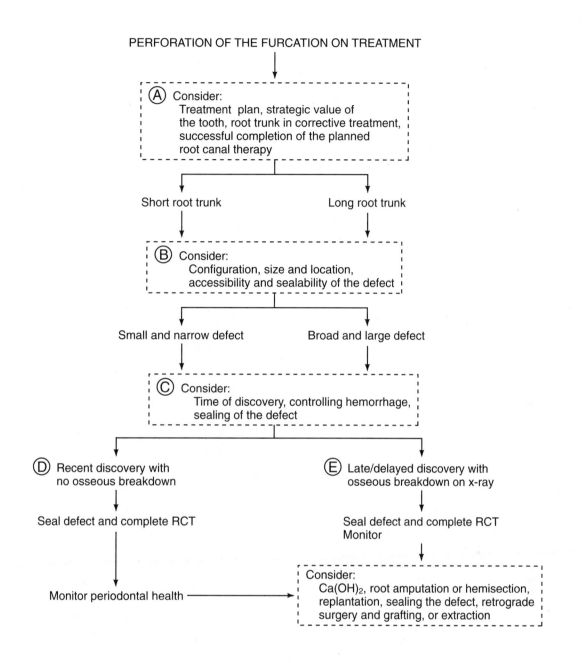

References

Bakland LK. Endodontic mishaps: Perforations. Calif Dent Assoc J 1991; 19(4):41.

Balla R, LoMonaco CJ, Skribner J, Lin LM. Histologic study of furcation perforations treated with tricalcium phosphate, hydroxylapatite, amalgam, and life. J Endodon 1991; 17(5):234.

Benenati FW, Roane JB, Biggs JT, Simon JH. Recall evaluation of iatrogenic root perforations repaired with amalgam and gutta-percha. J Endodon 1986; 12(4):161.

Harbert H: Generic tricalcium phosphate plugs: An adjunct in endodontics. J Endodon 1991; 17(3):131.

Ibarrola JL, Bjorenson JE, Austin BP, Gerstein H. Osseous reactions to three hemostatic agents. J Endodon 1985; 11(2):75.

Roane JB, Benenati FW. Successful management of a perforated molar using amalgam and hydroxylapatite. J Endodon 1987; 13(8):400.

MANAGING THE PERFORATED ROOT ON SINGLE-ROOTED TEETH

William W. Y. Goon

An iatrogenic perforation of the single-rooted tooth can occur at any level of the root during endodontic and operative manipulations into or within the root canal space. Unexpected hemorrhaging and pain are the pathognomonic signs and symptoms heralding a perforation in the previously dry root canal of an asymptomatic tooth. The discussion that follows assumes that (1) completion of the planned endodontics is not problematic and (2) the periodontal supporting tissues are in optimum health.

A. Perforations of the root are generally categorized according to the level of the root which is involved. Access preparation into the tooth and canal-widening procedures can result in perforations at the coronal level. Postspace preparation and conceptual deficiencies in managing the curved canal can lead to perforations at midroot level. The unskilled use of endodontic instruments can result in perforation of the apical foramen or, laterally, through the side at the apex of the root.

B. The coronal perforation can be identified through direct visualization into the tooth or confirmed by a misaligned endodontic instrument seen on the radiograph. The coronal defect is labelled as either at the supracrestal, crestal, or subcrestal bone level. Orthograde accessibility to the defect is usually not problematic; however, the sealing of the defect can be difficult. Periodontal complications are inevitably seen with an ineffective seal of the defect or with gross extrusion of sealing materials into the periodontal supporting tissues.

C. An orthograde repair of the defect should be attempted for an area that is above or below the crestal bone level. With a large defect the root canal space is first blocked with a solid object such as a silver cone to ensure patency; this is followed by the circumferential insertion of repair materials such as amalgam, Cavit, IRM, or condensation of gutta-percha with sealer cement. Esthetic considerations and the need to surgically remove any extruded material determine the appropriate material to use.

D. Surgical crown lengthening can expeditiously expose the defect for external sealing or inclusion under full coronal crown coverage. A solid object blocking the root canal space can serve as a matrix against which the reparative materials can be condensed and insures reaccess into the root canal space. The procedure is indicated primarily for defects directly involving the crestal bone. Without crown lengthening osseous breakdown often results from the irritating effects of the sealing materials and proximity of the defect to sulcular epithelium.

Although crown lengthening is a definitive treatment for the involved root, coronal coverage on a narrower root trunk may result in a marginally esthetic or disproportionately longer clinical crown. Also, the loss of osseous tissue support can adversely affect the periodontal health of the adjacent teeth. Consideration of these outcomes is necessary before a procedure is selected. However, for the perforated abutment tooth under a bridge the only acceptable treatment option is to surgically expose and seal the defect, leaving a residual periodontal pocket upon healing. The prognosis for tooth retention is favorable.

E. Root extrusion is an option for exposing a defect that is inaccessible to a predictable orthograde repair or where crown lengthening is likely to compromise the periodontal support of the adjacent healthy root (teeth). The outcome of root extrusion must be viewed from the perspective of the involved root. Although root extrusion conserves the crestal bone level and maintains the periodontal support of adjacent teeth, the involved root loses root length and the result is a restoration with compromised esthetics because of a narrower root trunk. The prognosis for tooth retention is favorable.

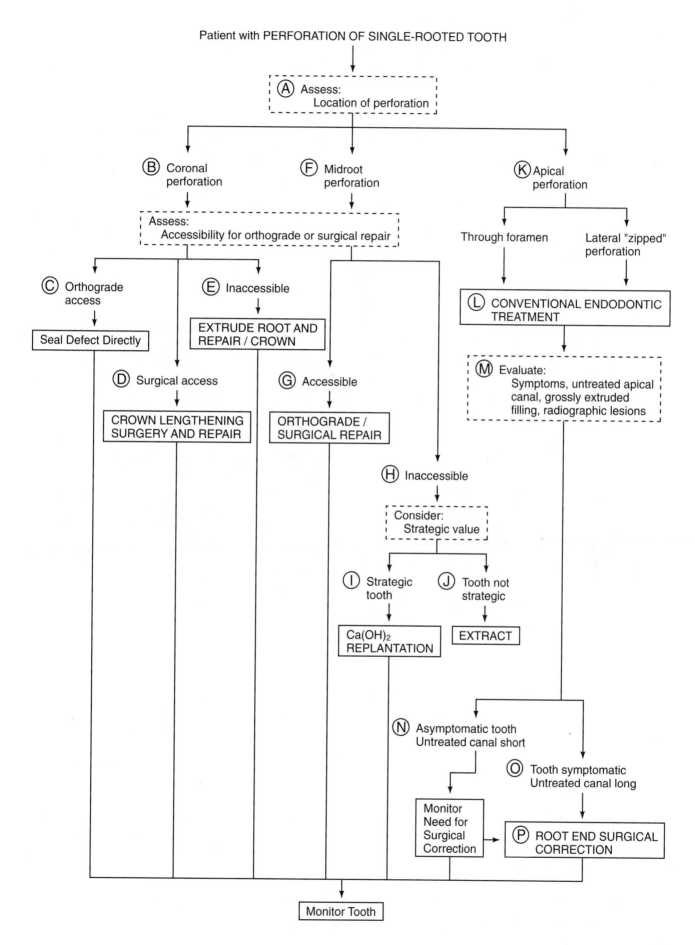

Patient with PERFORATION OF SINGLE-ROOTED TOOTH

Ⓐ Assess:
Location of perforation

Ⓑ Coronal
perforation

Ⓕ Midroot
perforation

Ⓚ Apical
perforation

Assess:
Accessibility for orthograde or surgical repair

Through foramen

Lateral "zipped"
perforation

Ⓒ Orthograde
access

Ⓔ Inaccessible

Ⓛ CONVENTIONAL ENDODONTIC
TREATMENT

Seal Defect Directly

EXTRUDE ROOT AND
REPAIR / CROWN

Ⓜ Evaluate:
Symptoms, untreated apical
canal, grossly extruded
filling, radiographic lesions

Ⓓ Surgical access

Ⓖ Accessible

CROWN LENGTHENING
SURGERY AND REPAIR

ORTHOGRADE /
SURGICAL REPAIR

Ⓗ Inaccessible

Consider:
Strategic value

Ⓘ Strategic
tooth

Ⓙ Tooth not
strategic

Ca(OH)₂
REPLANTATION

EXTRACT

Ⓝ Asymptomatic tooth
Untreated canal short

Ⓞ Tooth symptomatic
Untreated canal long

Monitor
Need for
Surgical
Correction

Ⓟ ROOT END SURGICAL
CORRECTION

Monitor Tooth

F. Midroot perforations typically occur during preparation of space for a post or intracanal widening procedures. Unexpected pain and hemorrhage and radiographic evidence of an overly wide post within a narrow root or a post that courses through the root eccentrically are pathognomonic of a perforation. Persistent postcementation sensitivity can also herald a perforation by the post that had exited through an invaginated area of the root. The defect is not readily apparent on the radiograph, which may demonstrate a properly aligned post.

G. A perforation on a post space preparation can be caused by overwidening of the canal space or the creation of an artificial channel that is skewed off the long axis of the root canal. In either event the defect is usually accessible for orthograde repair. A matrix constructed from calcium hydroxide, tricalcium phosphate, or Gelfoam may be required to control hemorrhage and provide a surface for condensation of amalgam or gutta-percha with sealer cement. A direct surgical repair may be used in labial/buccal perforations where the osseous matrix is too thin or is completely destroyed. The potential for vestibular soft tissue discoloration may warrant the sealing of the defect with a nonstaining material like Super EBA or IRM, especially in the anterior regions of the mouth. Treatment options for the post-restored perforated root is limited by the surgical approach and accessibility.

H. Aggressive or uncontrolled endodontic preparation can result in a large perforation through the lateral aspect of the root. In the single-rooted tooth, a lateral perforation is identical to a "stripped perforation" seen in the multirooted tooth. Accessibility to the midroot level is difficult, and control of hemorrhaging can be problematic. The practical management of this mishap rests primarily on the strategic value of the tooth and whether the hemorrhaging can be controlled to permit the uncontaminated sealing of the entire root canal space.

I. For the strategic tooth, treatment options may involve a prolonged and persistent attempt at using calcium hydroxide to control hemorrhaging or to induce the formation of an osseous barrier for condensation of sealing materials. Even with an osseous barrier the weakened condition of the root may predispose it to further treatment complications of root fracture on sealing procedures. Intentional replantation following the extraoral sealing of the defect may offer a more expeditious result but with attendant root complications of fracture or resorption. The prognosis for tooth retention is guarded.

J. A tooth is deemed nonsalvageable if the defect is extensive, lacks a barrier matrix, cannot be adequately sealed by orthograde or surgical methods, has a weakened root, or cannot be managed without compromising the periodontal support around it and the adjacent teeth. The tooth should be extracted under these circumstances.

K. An apical perforation sometimes is discovered on the radiograph(s) at the completion of root canal preparation. Perforation through the foramen is the most common mishap seen in the canal that is relatively straight. The perforation can also occur laterally alongside of the foramen. This mishap is referred to as a *zipped perforation,* a transported foramen, or an apical tear or rip on the surface of the root. Both mishaps result from inexperience and inability to (1) maintain the working length between successive enlarging instruments and (2) control the penetration of each instrument within the confines of the canal terminus. Additionally, the frequency and severity of the zipped perforation are functions of the degree of root curvature and canal curvature. The defect, formed with overextended instruments, is seen in the curved canal as a result of (1) failure to properly bend and rebend the instruments throughout preparation, (2) forceful insertion of rigid instruments into an underprepared canal, and (3) deliberate rotation of fragile or weakened instruments within the canal space.

L. Management of the apical perforation requires renegotiation of the canal, reestablishment of the correct length, and repair and sealing of the original canal space. For the curved canal that cannot be reentered, the instrument is withdrawn and preparation and sealing are confined to within the radiographic housing of the root. Extrusion of sealing material can be controlled by first constructing a barrier matrix by packing calcium hydroxide, tricalcium phosphate, or hydroxylapatite against the periapical tissues.

M. The prognosis in apical perforations is adversely affected by (1) inability to seal the defect and apex from leakage, (2) extrusion of sealing materials into the periapical tissues, and, in the curved root or canal, (3) the length of the untreated original apical canal space.

N. The tooth that remains asymptomatic and has no radiographic evidence of periapical breakdown should be monitored. This includes all teeth regardless of the result of the sealing procedure (filled adequately, overextended, or underextended).

O. The tooth that is causing the patient severe discomfort or pain, is grossly overfilled, or radiographically demonstrates a periapical lesion should be considered for definitive surgical correction.

P. The prognosis for tooth retention following surgical correction of the perforated apex is favorable. Postsurgical root-to-crown ratio should be 1:1 or greater. For a strategic tooth with poor periodontal osseous support, intentional replantation and extraoral sealing of the defect may conserve root length and salvage the tooth; however, postreplantation complications can result in a guarded-to-poor prognosis for the tooth.

References

Bakland LK. Endodontic mishaps: Perforations. Calif Dent Assoc J 1991; 19:41.

Ingle JI, Abou-Rass M. Perforations and their management. In: Ingle JI, Taintor JF, eds. Endodontics. 3rd ed. Philadelphia: Lea & Febiger, 1985:776.

Oswald RJ. Procedural accidents and their repair. Dent Clin North Am 1979; 23:593.

Torabinejad M: Endodontic mishaps: Etiology, prevention, and management. Alpha Omegan 1990; 83:42.

Webber RT: Iatrogenic root perforations. In: Gerstein H, ed. Techniques in clinical endodontics. Philadelphia: WB Saunders, 1983:185.

CONVENTIONAL VERSUS SURGICAL ENDODONTICS

Joseph H. Schulz

Whether pulpal pathosis is confined within tooth structure or spreads into the periodontal tissue and alveolar bone, a tooth that is proven to be nonvital is a candidate for endodontic therapy. *Conventional endodontics* consists of thorough pulp removal, shaping of the root canal system, and sealing the debrided space to prevent toxic by-products of cellular degeneration from irritating the vital tissues of the alveolar housing. *Surgical endodontics* is an alternative to be used sparingly and only in those cases where conventional therapy cannot be done or has not been successful. Root end resection and root end filling are the basis of surgical endodontics. No existing seal is effective for a lifetime. Accessory canals can also enable products of pulpal degeneration to gain access to the alveolus, conventional endodontics therefore has a greater chance of long-term success than does the surgical approach.

A. Once the tooth has been diagnosed as nonvital, the patency of the canal from the pulp chamber to the apex must be assessed. If it is patent, conventional endodontics should be performed prior to restoration.

B. If it is not patent to the apex because of calcifications, severe curvatures that cannot be negotiated, instrumentation accidents, obstructions, perforations, or apical root fractures, then surgical endodontics should be performed after debridement and the sealing of the pulp space as close to the apex as possible.

C. If the tooth has been restored previously, determine whether the restoration can be removed without damaging the structural integrity of the root. If so, conventional endodontics should be employed.

D. If the existing restoration cannot be removed safely (e.g., postcrown), surgical endodontics is indicated.

E. If an existing endodontic procedure is failing, retreatment should be considered. If there are no compromising factors (e.g., root fracture or perforation) and the canals appear accessible for instrumentation, conventional endodontics is the retreatment choice.

F. If retreatment does not seem promising to improving the conventional results, surgical endodontics should be considered.

G. If conventional retreatment or the surgical approach is failing, extraction must be considered.

References

Cohen S, Burns R. Pathways of the pulp. 5th ed. St Louis: Mosby–Year Book, 1991:166.

Guttman JL, Harrison JW. Surgical endodontics. Boston: Blackwell Scientific Publications, 1991:3.

Lovdahl PE. Dent Clin North Am 1992; 36(2):473.

Seltzer S. Endodontic retreatment. Endodontology: biologic considerations in endodontic procedures. Philadelphia: Lea & Febiger, 1988:439.

Walton RE, Torabinejad M. Principles and practice of endodontics. Philadelphia: WB Saunders, 1989:295.

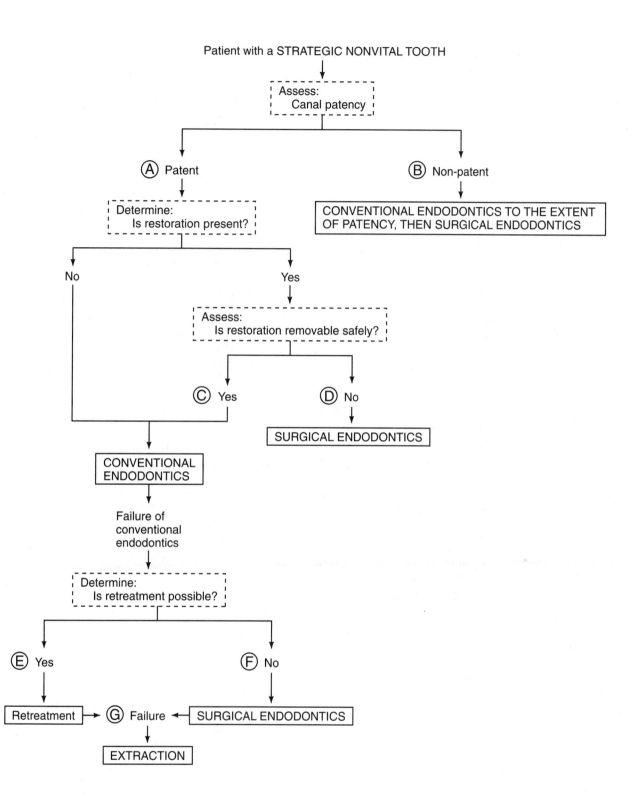

Patient with a STRATEGIC NONVITAL TOOTH

Assess:
Canal patency

(A) Patent

(B) Non-patent

Determine:
Is restoration present?

CONVENTIONAL ENDODONTICS TO THE EXTENT OF PATENCY, THEN SURGICAL ENDODONTICS

No

Yes

Assess:
Is restoration removable safely?

(C) Yes

(D) No

SURGICAL ENDODONTICS

CONVENTIONAL ENDODONTICS

Failure of conventional endodontics

Determine:
Is retreatment possible?

(E) Yes

(F) No

Retreatment → (G) Failure ← SURGICAL ENDODONTICS

EXTRACTION

RETREATMENT VERSUS SURGICAL ENDODONTICS FOR A SYMPTOMATIC, ENDODONTICALLY TREATED TOOTH

Borja Zabelegui

When a previously treated endodontic tooth is symptomatic, the dentist must decide whether retreatment or surgical endodontics (apicoectomy) is indicated if the tooth is important in the overall treatment plan.

A. If upon clinical examination the tooth is symptomatic (presents with spontaneous pain or pain to percussion), has a fistula or is suppurating, or has a periapical radiolucency that has increased in size following root canal therapy, failure of the earlier endodontics should be suspected.

B. The dentist must decide whether retreatment is indicated and is possible to perform. Unless better obturation appears impossible because of calcification or tortuosity of the canal(s), retreatment should be attempted with the patient fully informed of possible complications and the probability of success.

C. Intracoronal access should be attempted. If a post is present, it must be removed. The canal(s) should be thoroughly debrided, and shaped for placement of new filling material. If this can be completed successfully after the appropriate healing period, restoration can be performed.

   If retreatment cannot be completed and/or signs and symptoms of the earlier failure persist, surgical endodontics (apicoectomy) is indicated.

D. In those cases for which the dentist decides that retreatment cannot be performed or in which retreatment is unsuccessful, surgical access should be created.

E. If surgical access indicates that apicoectomy is feasible, it should be performed and the tooth restored after the appropriate healing period. If surgical access indicates that apicoectomy cannot be performed (e.g., because of fused roots) or is not indicated as a result of complicating factors (e.g., previously undetected cracks extending throughout the roots), either the tooth should be extracted or replantation might be considered despite the limited success of this procedure.

References

Arens DE. Surgical endodontics. In: Cohen S, Burns RC, eds. Pathways of the pulp. 5th ed. St Louis: Mosby–Year Book, 1991:574.

Frank AC, Weine FS. Non-surgical therapy for the perforative defect of internal resorption. J Am Dent Assoc 1973; 87:863.

Friedman S, Stabholz A. Endodontic treatment: Case selection and technique. 1. Criteria for case selection. J. Endodon 1986; 12:28.

Pitts DL, Natkin E. Diagnosis and treatment of vertical root fracture. J Endodon 1983; 9:338.

Stabholz A, Friedman S, Tamse A. Endodontic failures and retreatment. In: Cohen S, Burns RC, eds. Pathways of the pulp. 5th ed. St Louis, Mosby, 1991:752.

Patient with an IMPORTANT, SYMPTOMATIC, PREVIOUSLY ENDODONTICALLY TREATED TOOTH

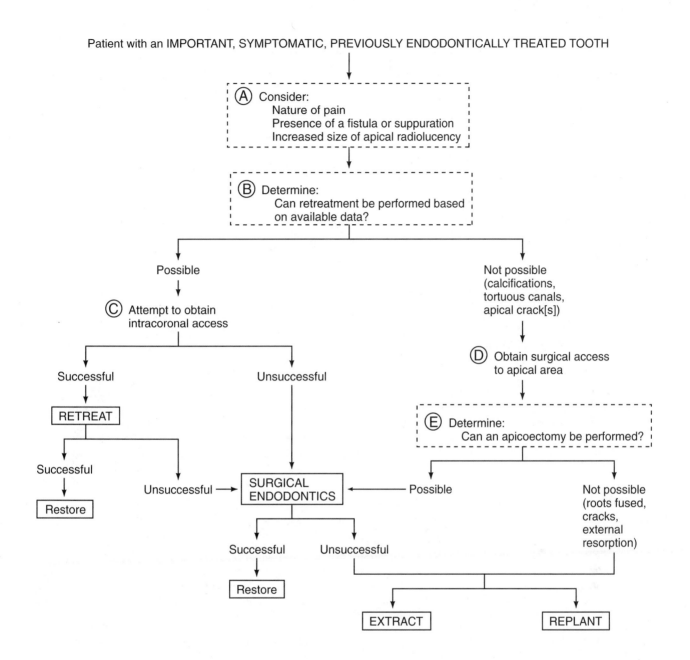

INDICATIONS FOR MOLAR TOOTH RADISECTION: HEMISECTION VERSUS ROOT AMPUTATION

Jordi J. Cambra
Borja Zabelegui

Root radisection is a technique for maintaining a portion of a diseased or injured molar by removal of one or more of its roots. Radisection may be achieved by hemisection, in which the entire tooth is cut in half and one part is removed, or by root amputation, in which only one or two roots are amputated from the remainder of the tooth (Fig. 1). These surgical approaches may be useful in many situations. The indications for selecting hemisection or root amputation depend on the status of the individual molar and its relationship to other teeth. Guided tissue regeneration may be a viable option instead of radisection (see p 62).

A. If a molar has fused roots, neither hemisection nor root amputation is possible. If a Class II furcation is present (see p 60), guided tissue regeneration may be attempted. If a Class III furcation is present (see p 58), extraction or maintenance with a hopeless prognosis can be done.

B. A maxillary molar with advanced involvement of a proximal furcation and separated roots where adjacent root proximity is a problem is treated by root amputation to facilitate access for debridement by the dentist and the patient. Where root proximity is not a complicating factor, a Class II (definite) furcation involvement proximally could be treated by guided tissue regeneration or mucogingival-osseous surgery or maintained with frequent planing (see p 30). The patient could enhance plaque control with an interproximal brush. The same is true when the facial furcation has a Class II involvement; however, if the furcations join one another (Class III), root amputation is indicated.

C. A mandibular molar with advanced furcation involvement and separated roots that is an existing bridge abutment is a candidate for root amputation and retention of the existing bridge; a similarly involved mandibular molar that is not an existing bridge abutment is treated by hemisection and crowning. In either case, if a Class II furcation is involved, guided tissue regeneration may be attempted. If a Class III furcation is present, hemisection or root amputation (if the tooth is part of an existing bridge) should be performed.

D. If there is no endodontic involvement, periodontal considerations become of paramount importance. The roots to be amputated must be determined. If the root to be removed is clearly indicated, endodontics should be done before amputation; if there is a doubt, surgery and vital root amputation allow for clinical decisions to be made. If the molar is mandibular and is an abutment for an existing fixed bridge, root amputation may permit retention of that bridge. If it is not an existing abutment, hemisection and then crowning are indicated.

E. When a necrotic pulp condition exists, endodontic treatment should be done prior to periodontal treatment. The differential diagnosis becomes difficult when the bone loss causing a deep pocket formation may be related to the failure of the root canal therapy as a result of technical errors (poor obturations). Perforations or vertical root fracture with no separation of fragments may cause bone loss defects that can mask primary periodontal conditions.

F. If the molar being considered has a cracked or perforated root, part of it may be salvaged by radisection. If the tooth is asymptomatic, either maintenance with a guarded prognosis may be considered or a surgical approach could be used. If the tooth is symptomatic and not of strategic (long-term) value, it may be extracted; however, if the tooth has strategic value, it should be treated. If the tooth is mandibular and is an abutment for an existing bridge, root amputation should be considered if root canal therapy can be performed on the root to be retained. If it is not an abutment for an existing bridge, hemisection is a better option. If the molar is maxillary and a single facial root is cracked or perforated, root amputation is indicated if root canal therapy can be performed on remaining roots. If both facial roots are cracked or perforated, root amputation with removal of both facial roots is a reasonable choice.

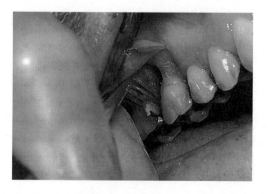

Figure 1. The distal facial root of this first molar has been resected and is being withdrawn from the socket.

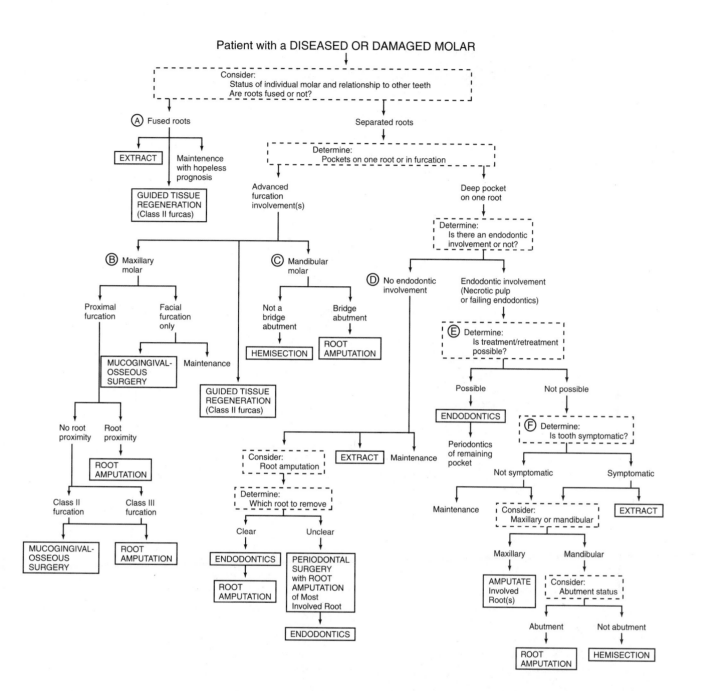

Patient with a DISEASED OR DAMAGED MOLAR

References

Amen CR. Hemisection and root amputation. Periodontics 1966; 4:197.

Basaraba N. Root amputation and tooth hemisection. Dent Clin North Am 1969; 13:121.

Grant DA, Stern IB, Listgarten MA. Periodontics. 6th ed. St Louis: CV Mosby, 1988:935.

Hiatt WH, Owen CR. Periodontal pocket elimination by combined therapy. Dent Clin North Am 1964; 8:133.

Schluger S, Yuodelis RA, Page RC, Johnson RH. Periodontal diseases. 2nd ed. Philadelphia: Lea & Febiger, 1990:548.

SEQUENCING ENDODONTICS AND ROOT RADISECTION

Jordi J. Cambra
Borja Zabelegui

When a patient has a tooth requiring combined endodontic and periodontal treatment (root radisection), the sequencing of the treatment requires considerable thought. Whenever possible, endodontic treatment should be done prior to root radisection to avoid difficulty in obtaining adequate anesthesia for comfortable root canal therapy, which could complicate endodontics following vital root resection. Vital root resection rarely results in serious postoperative pain; however, as degeneration of the exposed pulp progresses, increasing acidity interferes with the efficacy of the local anesthetic.

A. In a nonvital tooth the problem may be only endodontic, even when probing suggests deep pockets are present; this is especially true if the problem is severe and acute. If this appears to be the case, endodontics should be done first, as root radisection may not be needed if pockets no longer can be probed.

B. If root removal is needed, the first consideration is whether the roots to be resected are fused (Fig. 1). If so, the tooth must be extracted or maintained with a hopeless prognosis.

C. If the roots to be amputated are not fused, the dentist must decide whether or not to perform root canal therapy on all roots. If an untreatable root would be retained, the tooth should be extracted or maintained with a hopeless prognosis if symptom-free.

D. If endodontics can be done on all roots (or on all roots to be retained), determine which roots are to be resected. If doubt exists, periodontal surgery with vital resection of the root selected during surgery should be performed prior to endodontic treatment. If the roots to be amputated are clearly indicated, endodontic treatment should precede nonvital root radisection.

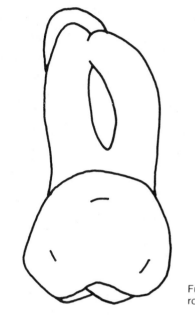

Fused roots

Figure 1. Roots that are fused at their apices are not candidates for root amputation.

References

Basaraba N. Root amputation and tooth hemisection. Dent Clin North Am 1969; 13:121.

Grant DA, Stern IB, Listgarten MA. Periodontics. 6th ed. St Louis: CV Mosby, 1988:916.

Hiatt WH, Amer CR. Periodontal pocket elimination by combined therapy. Dent Clin North Am 1964; 8:133.

Schluger S, Yuodelis RA, Page RC, Johnson RH. Periodontal diseases. 2nd ed. Philadelphia: Lea & Febiger, 1990:549.

Simons HS, Glick DH, Frank AL. The relationship of endodontic-periodontic lesions. J Periodontol 1972; 43:202.

Patient with MOLAR REQUIRING ROOT RADISECTION

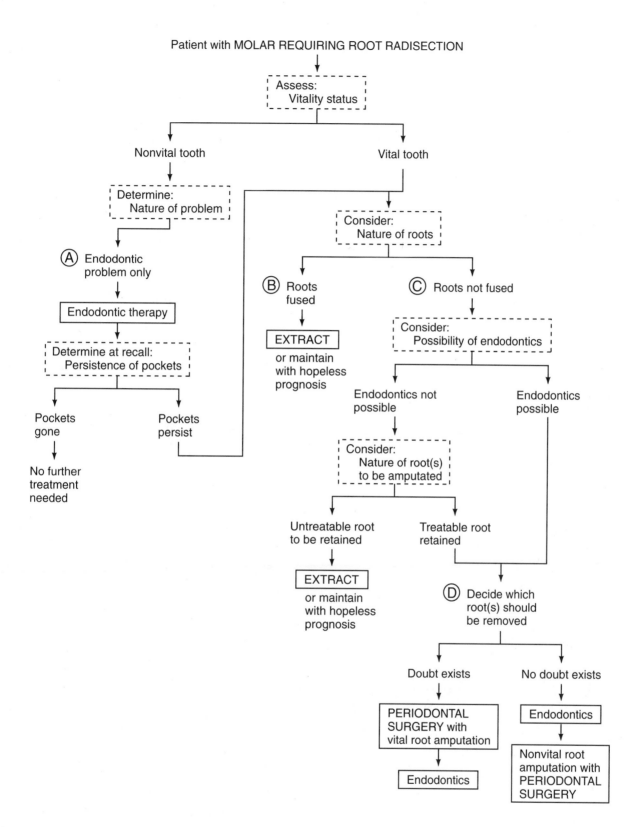

ROOT–END RESECTION AND ROOT–END FILLING: APICOECTOMY AND RETROGRADE FILLING

Joseph H. Schulz

Whenever conventional endodontics is failing or is considered impossible, the use of surgical endodontics must be considered if retention of the tooth is critical. Necrotic pulp by-products are a site for bacterial growth and, when they escape from within the root, can cause inflammation in the alveolar housing. The failure of conventional therapy causes symptoms or pathoses to persist or develop over time.

Root end resection (apicoectomy) is often employed to remove the source of the inflammation (terminal branchings), allow curettage of the diseased area, and provide access to the site that must be sealed. If endodontic surgery compromises the crown-to-root ratio or is likely to result in a secondary endodontic-periodontal lesion, the prognosis may be adversely affected and extraction may be the better choice.

To prevent future injury to the alveolar housing, a root end (retrograde) filling seals the toxic by-products within the root. All accessible portals of exit should be sealed from the root canal system during surgical endodontic procedures.

A. After the conventional endodontic approaches have been exhausted and there is persistence of periapical symptoms or the development of a lesion, surgical endodontics must be considered to retain a strategic tooth.

B. If an existing periodontal condition has resulted in crestal bone loss, the dentist must evaluate whether sufficient bone would remain after surgical endodontics. An endodontic-periodontal lesion could dramatically worsen the prognosis.

C. If surgical endodontics is required to seal a root surface near the gingival attachment, making the development of an unmanageable secondary endodontic-periodontal lesion likely, extraction should be considered.

D. If the crown-to-root ratio would be compromised by surgical endodontics (e.g., to eliminate a severe curvature or to seal an apical perforation), the dentist might consider extraction.

E. If the crown-to-root ratio is severely compromised by surgical endodontics and the tooth will be subjected to heavy occlusal forces, extraction should be considered.

F. A root end filling is recommended following all root end resection procedures. If this cannot be done and the conventional endodontics is inadequate, extraction should be recommended.

References

Dykema RW, et al: Johnston's modern practice in fixed prosthodontics. 4th ed. Philadelphia: WB Saunders, 1986:1.

Gartner AH, Dorn SO. Advances in endodontic surgery. Dent Clin North Am 1992; 36(2):357.

Guttman JL, Harrison JW. Surgical endodontics. Boston: Blackwell Scientific Publications, 1991:203, 338.

Pitts DL, Natkin E. Diagnosis and treatment of vertical root fractures. J Endodon 1983; 9(8):338.

Rapp EI, et al. An analysis of success and failure in apicoectomies. J Endodon 1991; 17(10):508.

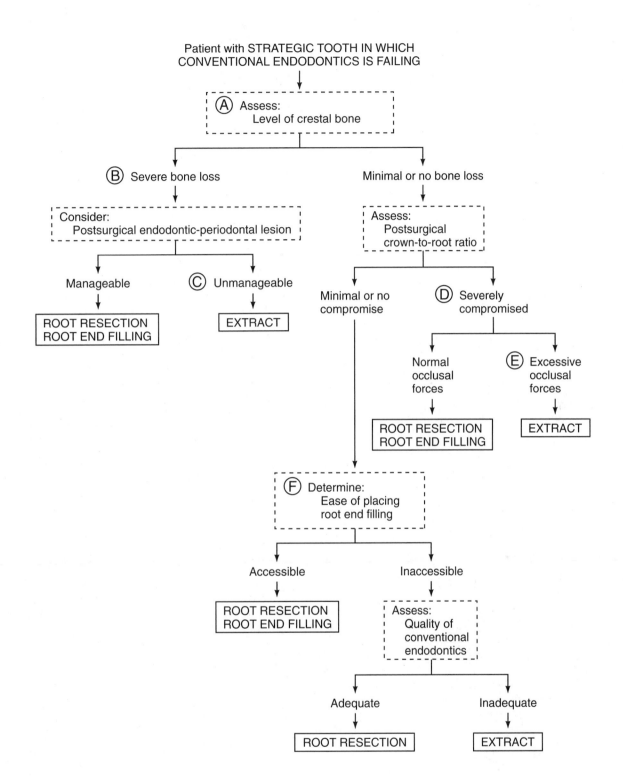

Patient with STRATEGIC TOOTH IN WHICH CONVENTIONAL ENDODONTICS IS FAILING

Ⓐ Assess:
Level of crestal bone

Ⓑ Severe bone loss

Minimal or no bone loss

Consider:
Postsurgical endodontic-periodontal lesion

Assess:
Postsurgical crown-to-root ratio

Manageable

Ⓒ Unmanageable

Minimal or no compromise

Ⓓ Severely compromised

ROOT RESECTION
ROOT END FILLING

EXTRACT

Normal occlusal forces

Ⓔ Excessive occlusal forces

ROOT RESECTION
ROOT END FILLING

EXTRACT

Ⓕ Determine:
Ease of placing root end filling

Accessible

Inaccessible

ROOT RESECTION
ROOT END FILLING

Assess:
Quality of conventional endodontics

Adequate

Inadequate

ROOT RESECTION

EXTRACT

RESTORATIVE PLANNING FOR ENDODONTICALLY TREATED POSTERIOR TEETH

W. Paul Brown
Arun Nayyar

For restorative management of a tooth that has undergone root canal therapy, clinical reevaluation of remaining tooth structure is needed. Tooth strength is greatly affected by the volume of intact tooth structure remaining after root canal treatment; thus it is imperative to minimize dentin removal. An endodontically treated tooth with a minimal access opening can be sealed with an amalgam or acid-etched composite resin. Most endodontically treated posterior teeth have lost one or both marginal ridges, and the access opening interrupts the integrity of the remaining dentin and enamel. Consequently, tooth strength, which had been provided by dentin and enamel, must be judiciously replaced. When a large volume of existing tooth structure has been lost, the restorative objective is to reinforce the remaining tooth structure to resist occlusal forces. This can be accomplished by a coronal radicular buildup, which provides needed retention and resistance form for the cast crown restoration.

A. In deciding whether an endodontically involved posterior tooth can be saved, such factors as the extensiveness of caries, the nature and extent of cracks or fractures, the periodontal and combined periodontal-endodontic nature of the pathology, and the need for crown lengthening or for orthodontic forced eruption must be weighed. Before proceeding, decide whether the tooth can be restored once endodontics is done or redone.

B. If the tooth can be treated endodontically and restoratively, a decision on the design of the restoration should be made. The amalgam dowel core buildup technique utilizes the pulp chamber for retention of the dowel and core segments. Most pulp chamber spaces are large enough to provide needed internal retention for the amalgam alloy.

   Amalgam condensed against dentin has structural strength and margin-sealing ability and is one of the easiest materials to use, requiring no special setup. The less substantial the clinical crown, the greater the retention the alloy requires. This needed retention usually can be obtained by using the pulp chamber and, in those instances when the pulp chamber walls are minimal or missing, 2 to 4 mm of the diverging root canal space. A conservative approach to gain retention is critical. The removal of any healthy dentin greatly weakens the remaining structures and directly affects the life of the final restoration. Slow setting time for amalgam can be accelerated by increasing the trituration time (Fig. 1).

   If an access opening is minimal, if endodontics is done through an existing crown, or if 20% or less of the clinical crown is missing, the amalgam dowel core can suffice as the final restoration.

C. If 40% to 80% of the clinical crown is missing, a cast crown is needed after an amalgam core buildup.

D. If 90% to 100% of the clinical crown is missing, a prefabricated or cast metal post can be employed to provide better retention of the buildup material. The placement of a post does not significantly improve the strength of the amalgam buildup. Additional dentin must be removed from the canal walls to permit post insertion, thus weakening the remaining tooth structure and increasing the likelihood of creating a crack or perforation. If crazing lines or near perforation indicate the need for better retention of the amalgam buildup, a resin liner may be employed to increase the adhesion of alloy to dentin. The use of resin to bond amalgam to dentin also permits the size of the preparation to be minimized (which would further decrease the likelihood of fracture). A cast crown should be utilized to complete the restoration.

E. If the tooth has been broken off at the gingival margin, a prefabricated cast dowel post may be employed to serve as a scaffold and amalgam condensed around it. A cast gold post is indicated only if there is access difficulty. A cast crown is utilized to complete the restoration. Whenever a cast crown is employed, its margins should reach 2 mm beyond the buildup material. Crown lengthening may be necessary to achieve this goal (see p 32).

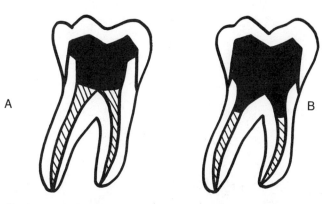

Figure 1. **A,** A pulp chamber greater than 3 mm in depth and/or with significant undercuts has adequate retention for a buildup. **B,** When pulp chamber characteristics do not provide adequate retention, extending the buildup into the canals can provide retention.

Patient with an ENDODONTICALLY INVOLVED POSTERIOR TOOTH THAT REQUIRES RESTORATION

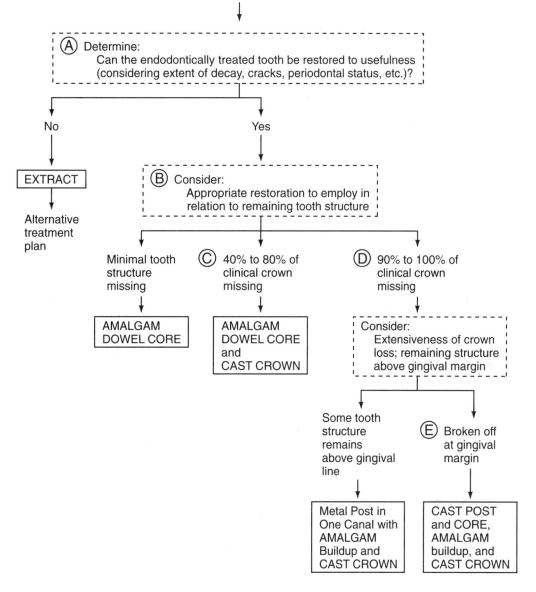

References

Kanca J. The all-etch bonded technique/wet bonding. Dent Today 1991; 18:57.

Lacy AM, Staninec MA. The bonded amalgam restoration. Quintessence Int 1989; 20:521.

Nayyar A. Coronal-radicular restorations (technique and materials). Clin Dent 1983; 4:1.

Radke RA, Eissmann HF. Postendodontic restoration. In: Cohen S, Burns RC, eds. Pathways of the pulp. 5th ed. St Louis: Mosby, 1991:640.

Staninec MA, Holt M. Bonding of amalgam to tooth structure: Tensile adhesion and microleakage tests. J Prosthet Dent 1988; 59:397.

Staninec M. Retention of amalgam restorations: Undercuts versus bonding. Quintessence Int 1989; 20:347.

INDICATIONS FOR THE TREATMENT
OF A VERTICALLY CRACKED TOOTH

Hipolito Fabra-Campos
Jose Manuel Roig-Garcia

A cracked tooth may have a longitudinal fracture at root level in an endodontically treated tooth. This fracture may extend from the root canal to the surrounding area, stretching along the length of the root either totally or partially. It may begin at the crown and continue along the length of the root towards the apex, or it may be localized along the root of the tooth with or without coronal effects.

Vertical root fractures can be caused by an excessive force produced within the root canal or in the pulp chamber as a result of root canal filling procedures, pin or post placement, seating of intracoronal restorations, or the reduction of the tooth's resistance following endodontic treatment.

A. If the endodontically treated tooth is painful, the cause should be determined. The presence of a cracked tooth can be suspected if a separation of the root or fissure lines exists or if a clear apex-lateral image or areas of external resorption are observed on x-ray. Surgical inspection is necessary if this diagnosis is not certain.

B. If there is no periodontal involvement and pain is present with or without an obvious periapical radiolucency, existing endodontics should be redone in case any contaminated pulp residue or unfilled canals are present. If the radiolucency is periapical, the fracture may be localized at the apex; thus, periapical surgery with retrofilling is indicated.

C. If there is periodontal involvement localized in a narrow infrabony pocket with limited depth in the surrounding area of the tooth, the prognosis is guarded because periodontal treatment is not a suitable solution for the lesion.

D. If the fracture is localized in the coronal third of the root, the deepest area of the pocket is situated at the apical limit of the fracture. Eliminate the fractured fragment and surgically expose or orthodontically extrude the remaining portion. Crown lengthening may be employed to expose the surrounding area of the root.

E. If the fracture extends along the length of the root or the tooth has a fused root, it may be possible to preserve it by eliminating debris from the interior of the canal and then filling with calcium hydroxide for a 9 to 12 month period. A full coverage temporary crown is indicated during this time. If after a few months the periodontal lesion disappears, the canal can be obturated with a fair prognosis. If time is not available, the tooth has no strategic value, or the periodontal damage does not resolve, extraction is indicated.

F. If the affected tooth is multirooted and the crack only affects one root, the indicated treatment in the case of separated roots is hemisection or amputation of the affected root. If a molar has fused roots and strategic value, temporary refilling using calcium hydroxide can be attempted. If the lesion does not disappear, extraction is indicated. If the fracture is in one or both of the facial roots of an upper molar, amputation or hemisection with removal of both facial roots are reasonable choices.

References

Ingle JI, Beveridge EF, eds. Endodontics. Philadelphia: Lea & Febiger, 1976:719.

Lin LM, Langeland K. Vertical root fracture. J Endodon 1982; 8:558.

Meister F, Lommel TJ, Gerstein H. Diagnosis and possible causes of vertical root fracture. Oral Surg 1980; 49:243.

Pitts DL, Natkin E. Diagnosis and treatment of vertical root fractures. J Endodon 1983; 9:338.

Polson AM. Periodontal destruction associated with vertical root fracture: Report of four cases. J Periodontol 1977; 48:27.

Stewart GG. The detection and treatment of vertical root fractures. J Endodon 1988; 14:47.

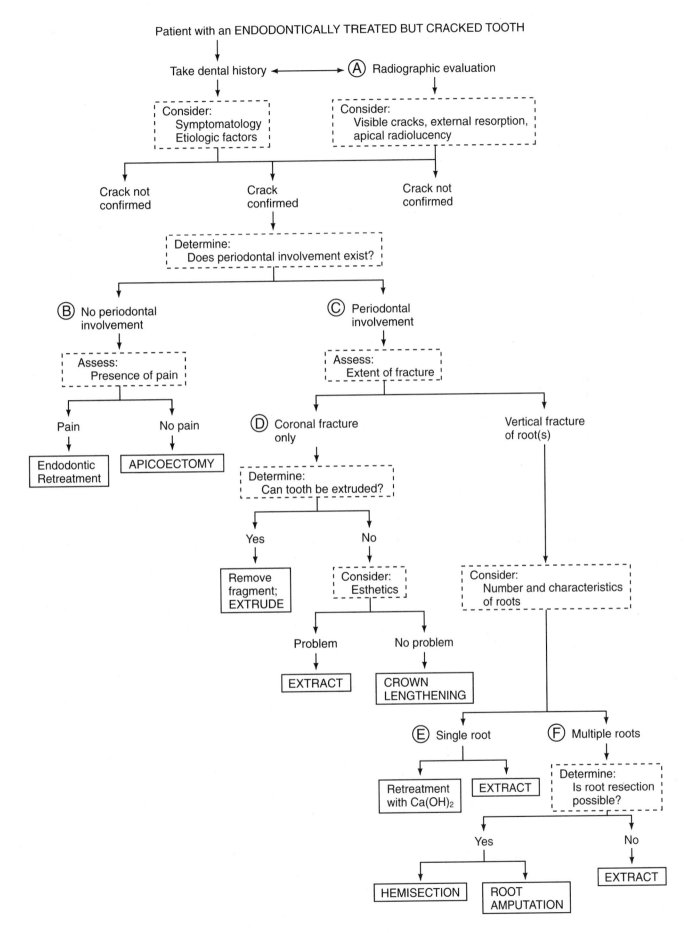

Patient with an ENDODONTICALLY TREATED BUT CRACKED TOOTH

Take dental history ←→ Ⓐ Radiographic evaluation

Consider:
    Symptomatology
    Etiologic factors

Consider:
    Visible cracks, external resorption,
    apical radiolucency

Crack not confirmed

Crack confirmed

Crack not confirmed

Determine:
    Does periodontal involvement exist?

Ⓑ No periodontal involvement

Ⓒ Periodontal involvement

Assess:
    Presence of pain

Assess:
    Extent of fracture

Pain

No pain

Ⓓ Coronal fracture only

Vertical fracture of root(s)

Endodontic Retreatment

APICOECTOMY

Determine:
    Can tooth be extruded?

Yes

No

Remove fragment; EXTRUDE

Consider:
    Esthetics

Consider:
    Number and characteristics of roots

Problem

No problem

EXTRACT

CROWN LENGTHENING

Ⓔ Single root

Ⓕ Multiple roots

Retreatment with Ca(OH)₂

EXTRACT

Determine:
    Is root resection possible?

Yes

No

HEMISECTION

ROOT AMPUTATION

EXTRACT

CLINICAL AND RADIOGRAPHIC CONSIDERATIONS PRIOR TO PLANNING ENDODONTICS IN COMPLEX CASES

Hipolito Fabra-Campos
Jose Manuel Roig-Garcia

In deciding whether a tooth merits endodontic treatment as part of an overall treatment plan, the amount of existing tooth structure remaining, its restorability, the existence of fractures, and, especially, its periodontal status must be determined before proceeding.

A.   Radiographic and clinical evaluation of the amount of tooth structure available and the adequacy of the remaining portion to support a restoration that is part of the overall treatment plan is the initial step. If the tooth is unrestorable (e.g., decay or tooth structure loss extends into a furcation, the remaining root structure is insufficient to support a crown), it should be extracted. If it is judged to be restorable, its endodontic status should be assessed.

B.   If the tooth is not endodontically involved, prosthetic preparation may necessitate pulpal exposure to meet demands for parallel abutment preparation or to reduce the crown height sufficiently to allow an adequate thickness of restorative material. If the pulp must be exposed to permit restoration of the tooth as an important part of the treatment plan, the possibility of performing root canal therapy should be assessed.

C.   Should the tooth appear to be fractured, the extent of the fracture(s) should be assessed. Fiberoptic and radiographic evaluation should be included in the decision regarding treatment options. A crack that is restricted to the crown should not influence the potential usefulness of the tooth. If the crack extends into the root and appears to involve only the coronal third, elimination of the coronal portion of the fracture may not endanger the continued usefulness of the tooth. Crown lengthening (see p 32) or orthodontic extrusion (see p 75) may permit its restoration. A more extensive fracture or a vertical fracture throughout the root would make the tooth unrestorable, and it should be extracted.

D.   The periodontal status of the tooth must be considered before proceeding with endodontic treatment. As attachment loss approaches 50%, the possibilities of successful periodontal treatment decline dramatically; however, the presence of periodontal lesions amenable to guided tissue regeneration (e.g., a deep three-walled osseous defect, a severe Class II furcation involvement, a deeper interdental crater) should not limit efforts to retain the tooth (see p 62). If the tooth is periodontally maintainable or can be made so, proceed with the indicated root canal therapy.

Should periodontal treatment result in a pulpal problem, a possible consequence of furcation surgery, proceed with endodontics, if feasible. With some molars root amputation or hemisection and endodontic treatment permit retention of strategically important parts of molars (see p 128).

E.   If all of the above considerations indicate that the tooth will be useful when endodontically treated, the feasibility of root canal therapy should be considered next. Access, internal and external resorption problems, unsatisfactory earlier root canal therapy, and other factors must be evaluated. When conventional endodontics cannot be employed, root resection or apicoectomy may permit retention of the tooth (see p 124). If these procedures cannot be performed or if they fail to be accomplished successfully, the tooth should be extracted.

References

Guilbert P, Rozanes SO, Tecuciano JF. Periodontal and prosthetic treatment of patients with advanced periodontal disease. Dent Clin North Am 1988; 32:331.

Kalwarf KL, Reinhardt RA. The furcation problem. Dent Clin North Am 1988; 32:243.

Lindhe J. Textbook of clinical periodontology. 2nd ed. Copenhagen: Munksgaard, 1989:569.

Nyman S, Lindhe J. A longitudinal study of combined periodontal and prosthetic treatment of patients with advanced periodontal disease. J Periodontol 1975; 50:163.

Trabert KC, Cooney JP. Endodontically treated teeth. Dent Clin North Am 1984; 28:923.

Patient with ENDODONTIC PROBLEM AND COMPLEX TREATMENT NEEDS

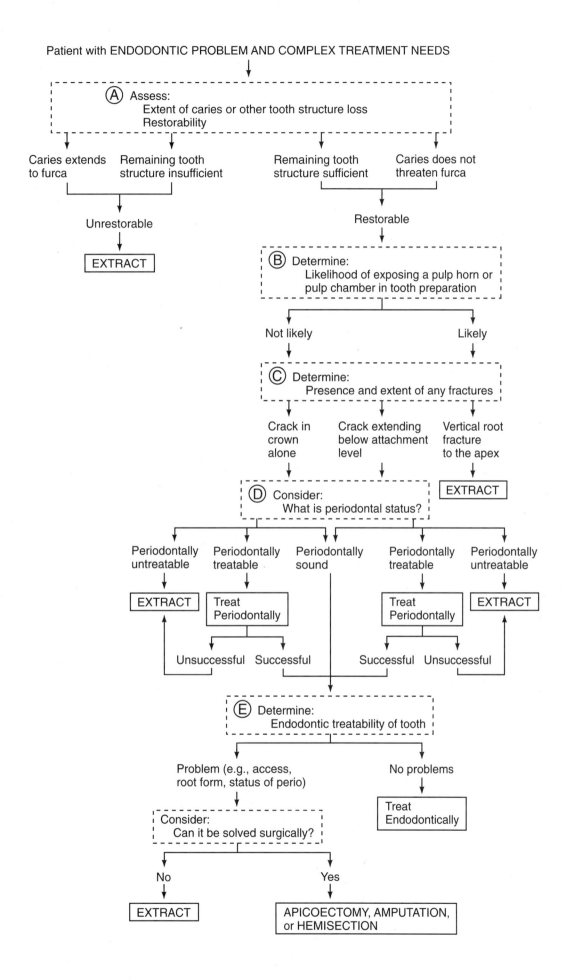

ORTHODONTICS

W. Eugene Roberts, Editor

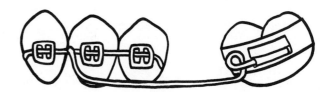

LIMITED ORTHODONTICS IN ADULTS

W. Eugene Roberts

Orthodontics is an increasingly important adjunct for maintaining and restoring adult occlusion. As the incidence of dental disease decreases, interest in comprehensive rehabilitation of the partially edentulous has increased. In many ways dentistry has entered the age of biomechanics. The emphasis is on managing the dental and musculoskeletal health of the entire stomatognathic system. Limited orthodontic therapy helps to salvage malaligned abutments or to stabilize periodontally compromised teeth. Rigid dental implants can serve as a source of firm orthodontic anchorage. In the context of modern practice, judicious orthodontics is an essential prerequisite for the dental rehabilitation of many partially edentulous patients.

A and B

Diagnosis. In addition to a routine health history, a specific assessment of bone metabolism is an important prerequisite to bone manipulative therapy. The major problem in considering orthodontics as an integral part of a comprehensive dentistry is appropriate diagnosis. All three planes (sagittal, horizontal [frontal], and vertical) must be considered. Because of the broad range of variability, there is no effective "cookbook approach" for orthodontic evaluation. Key issues for determining the complexity of the problem involve (1) the growing patient, (2) facial imbalance (convex, concave, or asymmetric), (3) lip protrusion or retrusion, (4) lip incompetence (>2 mm), (5) abnormal lip/tongue posture or habits, (6) dental crowding (>3 mm per arch), (7) >2 mm buccal interdigitation discrepancy (Class II or III), (8) overjet >3 mm, (9) overbite >50%, and (10) C_r to C_o discrepancy >1 mm.

In general, limited orthodontic problems amenable to management in general practice are nonskeletal (static) malocclusions in one plane. Most are dental alignment discrepancies such as dental crossbites, rotations, spacing, isolated crowding, and axial inclination of abutment roots. More experienced clinicians can manage problems involving two planes (i.e., where intrusion, extrusion, or arch width are superimposed on an alignment problem). However, malocclusions involving all three planes are challenging problems for orthodontists.

All dentists should develop skills to manage limited orthodontic problems. The decision as to what is truly "limited" requires far more training than the actual mechanics to accomplish treatment. Although the diagnostic process takes only a few minutes, the base of knowledge and experience from which an orthodontist draws is immense.

Treatment Planning. The prognostic ability to visualize a realistic result requires a thorough assessment of all orthodontic problems. It is important to avoid the temptation to formulate a treatment plan before an adequate diagnosis is made. Assuming an appropriate orthodontic screening, algorithms are provided in the following chapters for four common alignment problems: molar uprighting (p 144), nonrestorable space (p 150), flared incisors (p 152), and/or a fractured tooth (p 154). The flow charts are designed to assist in making specific diagnostic, referral, and treatment planning decisions.

Mechanics. In deciding to treat a limited orthodontic problem, remember that full archwires are difficult to control because they have a tendency to move all teeth. Correcting iatrogenic problems can be more challenging than treating the original malocclusion. The most effective mechanics for limited problems rely on extensive anchorage: cross-arch devices (lingual and palatal arches) in conjunction with well-focused segmental mechanics. Designs of specific appliances are illustrated in standard orthodontic texts. Less experienced clinicians are wise to seek the advice of an orthodontist. Most orthodontists are happy to help with a specific mechanics plan for a well defined problem.

References

Graber TM, Swain BF. Orthodontics: Current practice and techniques. St Louis: Mosby, 1985.

Hohlt WF, Roberts WE. Orthodontic education at Indiana University: A new philosophy of specialty and general practice. J Indiana Dent Assoc 1990; 69:19.

Proffit WR. Contemporary orthodontics. 2nd ed. St Louis: Mosby, 1993.

Roberts WE, Marshall KJ, Mozsary PG. Rigid endosseous implant utilized as anchorage to protract molars and close an atrophic extraction site. Angle Orthod 1990; 60:135.

Roberts WE, Simmons KE, Garetto LP, DeCastro RA. Bone physiology and metabolism in dental implantology: Risk factors for osteoporosis and other metabolic bone diseases. Implant Dent 1992; 1:11.

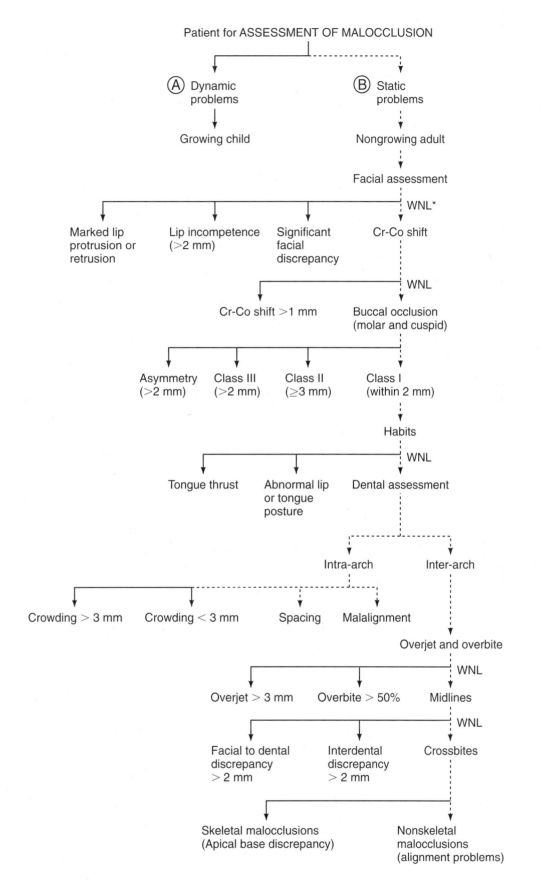

Patient for ASSESSMENT OF MALOCCLUSION

(A) Dynamic problems

(B) Static problems

Growing child

Nongrowing adult

Facial assessment

WNL*

Marked lip protrusion or retrusion

Lip incompetence (>2 mm)

Significant facial discrepancy

Cr-Co shift

WNL

Cr-Co shift >1 mm

Buccal occlusion (molar and cuspid)

Asymmetry (>2 mm)

Class III (>2 mm)

Class II (≥3 mm)

Class I (within 2 mm)

Habits

WNL

Tongue thrust

Abnormal lip or tongue posture

Dental assessment

Intra-arch

Inter-arch

Crowding > 3 mm

Crowding < 3 mm

Spacing

Malalignment

Overjet and overbite

WNL

Overjet > 3 mm

Overbite > 50%

Midlines

WNL

Facial to dental discrepancy > 2 mm

Interdental discrepancy > 2 mm

Crossbites

Skeletal malocclusions (Apical base discrepancy)

Nonskeletal malocclusions (alignment problems)

*WNL–Within Normal Limits
Dashed lines indicate within scope of general practice.

MOLAR UPRIGHTING/CREATING SPACE

Gordon R. Arbuckle

The tooth most often lost as a result of caries and or periodontal disease is the permanent first molar. Unless this condition is managed in a timely fashion, tipping, drifting, and rotation of the adjacent teeth will occur. Mesial tipping is usually the focus of attention, but correction of lingual inclination is of equal importance. Preprosthetic molar alignment is commonly indicated and can often be achieved with fixed orthodontic appliances. Careful periodontal and prosthodontic evaluation is essential before undertaking this orthodontic procedure. Orthodontic therapy in the presence of active periodontal disease can lead to rapid and irreversible deterioration of the periodontium. With careful diagnosis and treatment planning, this adjunctive procedure can significantly improve the final prosthetic restoration and create a periodontally manageable restored dentition.

A. Gingiva around tipped molars may appear pink, firm, and generally healthy; however, it may be fibrotic from repeated episodes of gingivitis. Inflammation may be present in the depths of the periodontal crevices. Therefore, probing of the gingival pockets is an essential part of the pretreatment evaluation. Orthodontic uprighting would be ill advised in the presence of active periodontal disease. Bleeding on probing is one of the most reliable indicators of inflammation. If no bleeding occurs and the pocket depths are within acceptable limits, inflammatory disease is absent or minimal. In the presence of bleeding, a comprehensive periodontal evaluation is needed.

B. Periodontitis is characterized clinically by a loss of attachment. If the probing depth is 0 to 3 mm with no loss of attachment and no bleeding noted on gentle probing, the gingiva may be assumed to be healthy and orthodontic treatment can be initiated. Pockets greater than 3 mm indicate the need for periodontal evaluation before and at regular intervals during orthodontic treatment. The periodontal treatment of choice for a prospective molar uprighting procedure is to maintain the area by nonsurgical means. If indicated, surgical procedures and more aggressive care should be accomplished 4 to 6 months prior to appliance placement.

C. The assessment of adequate attached gingiva varies considerably from tooth to tooth and even from surface to surface on the same tooth. It is a matter of clinical judgment as to the likelihood of a tooth remaining stable and healthy during an orthodontic procedure such as uprighting. It is suggested that areas with less than 2 mm of keratinized gingiva be considered as a potential problem because the resulting attached gingiva will probably be only 1 mm when the crevice depth is subtracted. Teeth having less than 1 mm of attached gingiva are potential candidates for grafting. These pretreatment decisions require full consideration of the potential additional insults that the orthodontic appliance, lack of accessibility for hygiene, and eruption of the tooth may cause.

D. The prognosis for orthodontically uprighting a molar with furcation involvement is guarded. In general, furcations are considered likely areas for recurrence of active bone loss from periodontitis. It is unwise to upright a molar and place a prosthesis in an area where the periodontium cannot be maintained. If an incipient furcation involvement is suspected, the patient should be referred for proper diagnosis, classification, and treatment. Furcation care is complex and requires regular periodontal maintenance during the orthodontic procedure.

E. If an edentulous space opposes the molar(s) to be uprighted, serious thought must be given as to the justification for an uprighting procedure. It is possible that either mesial or distal movement of the uprighted molar(s) may establish an opposing occlusion. Restoration of opposing edentulous areas requires a complete prosthetic evaluation and treatment plan.

F. If uprighting moves the tooth out of occlusion, a mesial-distal adjustment may be necessary to maintain contact with the opposing dentition. Such adjustments may be easily accomplished but often dictate the need for a more comprehensive course of orthodontic treatment.

G. Numerous techniques for molar uprighting and/or space closure have been presented in the literature. A typical segmental uprighting appliance is shown in Figure 1.

The primary mechanical consideration is that control of the vertical extrusion of an uprighted tooth requires significant anchorage requirements, and therefore bonding/banding of additional teeth is obviously necessary. Use of cross-arch stabilization via a lingual or transpalatal arch is often needed.

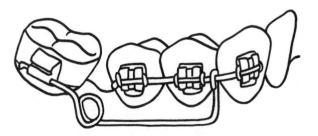

Figure 1 Typical segmental uprighting appliance.

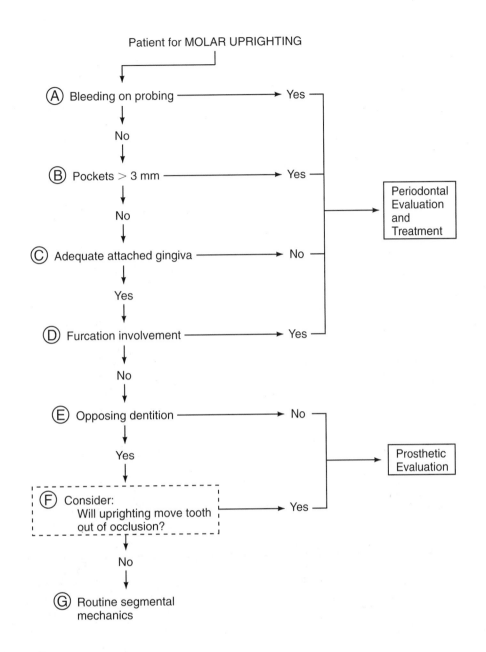

Patient for MOLAR UPRIGHTING

(A) Bleeding on probing ——————→ Yes

No

(B) Pockets > 3 mm ——————→ Yes

No

(C) Adequate attached gingiva ——————→ No

Yes

(D) Furcation involvement ——————→ Yes

Periodontal
Evaluation
and
Treatment

No

(E) Opposing dentition ——————→ No

Yes

(F) Consider:
    Will uprighting move tooth
    out of occlusion? ——————→ Yes

Prosthetic
Evaluation

No

(G) Routine segmental
    mechanics

References

Hall WB. Decision making in periodontology. Philadelphia: BC Decker, 1988.

Moyers RE. Handbook of orthodontics. 4th ed. Chicago: Year Book Medical Publishers, 1988.

Proffit WR. Contemporary orthodontics. 2nd ed. St Louis: Mosby, 1993:558-569.

Roberts WE, Marshall KJ, Mozsary PG. Rigid endosseous implant utilized as anchorage to protract molars and close an atrophic extraction site. Angle Orthod 1990; 60:135.

MANAGEMENT OF EDENTULOUS SPACE IN THE LOWER POSTERIOR SEGMENT

W. Eugene Roberts

Because of the decline in the incidence of caries and periodontal disease, an increasing segment of the population is partially edentulous but otherwise dentally healthy. Recent epidemiologic studies document that a common problem is isolated loss of the first or second mandibular molar as a result of caries in childhood or adolescence. Optimal restoration in affected patients is a challenging problem because of malaligned abutments, extrusion of occlusal antagonists, heavy occlusal loading in the molar regions, and long-term hygiene problems associated with fixed prostheses. Many patients benefit from preprosthetic alignment of abutments and occlusal antagonists. For some patients orthodontic space closure is a viable consideration.

Many patients with posterior missing teeth are young adults. Based on life expectancy, the functional service requirement is usually more than 50 years. Because of mechanical, secondary caries, and periodontal problems, routine fixed bridges are serviceable for only about 10 to 12 years. Replacing a fixed prosthesis is often a challenging and expensive problem because of abutment and periodontal deterioration. If a natural tooth is available to close the space, orthodontics is usually superior to a series of increasingly compromised prostheses.

Treatment options for management of an isolated lower first molar extraction site include (1) three-unit fixed bridge, (2) implant with a single tooth replacement crown, and (3) orthodontic space closure. A removable partial denture for restoration of a lower first molar extraction site is rarely indicated. In most cases orthodontic space closure is a viable option only when the third molar is present or the upper second and third molars are missing. Because of heavy loading and hygiene problems over a lifetime, the orthodontic solution is functionally superior to prosthetics. However, orthodontics takes longer because the rate of translation for lower molars is only about 0.3 mm per month. Closing a molar extraction site usually requires from 24 to 30 months. The major advantage is that orthodontics is usually a permanent solution to the problem compared to the <20 years service expected from most implant-supported or fixed prostheses.

A. Adequacy of the dentition distal to the first or second molar extraction site is the initial consideration. Assuming upper first and second molars are present and in Class I occlusion, an adequate third molar on the affected side is essential for an optimal orthodontic result. The key diagnostic questions are: Is the third molar present? If so, is it accessible for orthodontics? If not, is it salvageable by uncovering, uprighting, and/or repositioning? In the absence of an adequate third molar, implant-supported or conventional prosthodontics to restore the missing molar is indicated. If upper second and third molars are missing, moving the second molar mesially to close a first molar extraction site is a good option.

B. Adequate anchorage for conventional orthodontic space closure is the next consideration. Because molar spaces are usually ≥10 mm, it is rarely possible to close the space without an unacceptable skewing of the arch. In the exceptional circumstance that adequate anchorage is available, conventional orthodontics is indicated. In the absence of adequate anchorage, an orthodontically dedicated implant is a viable option.

C. An adequate site for placing the implant outside the arch is the next consideration. The implant is usually placed on the retromolar slope of the alveolar process about 5 mm distal to the third molar; however, it is possible to utilize the medial aspect of the external oblique ridge as an alternative site. In the absence of an adequate site outside the arch, complete space closure is not possible if the implant is placed in the extraction site. On the other hand, some mesial movement of molars may be accomplished by placing the implant as far mesial as possible in the edentulous area.

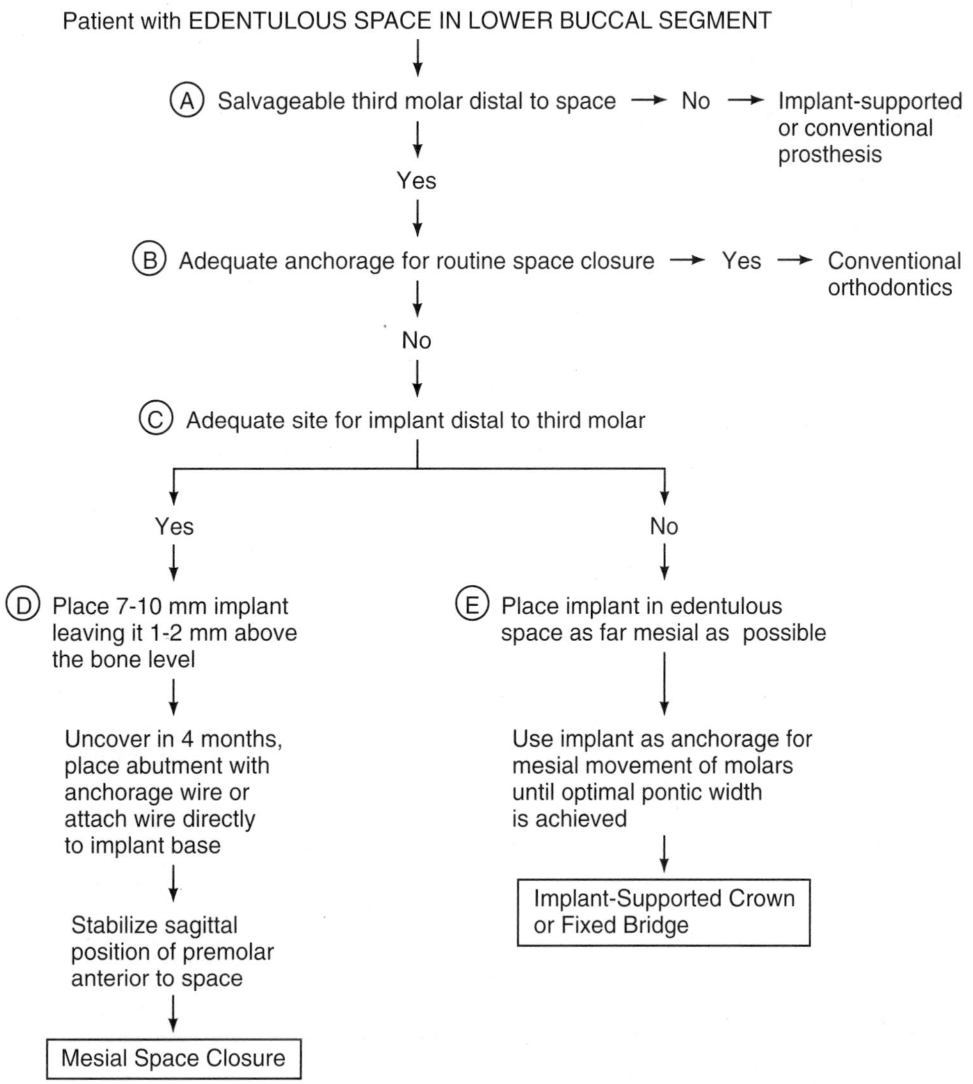

Patient with EDENTULOUS SPACE IN LOWER BUCCAL SEGMENT

⏷

Ⓐ Salvageable third molar distal to space ⟶ No ⟶ Implant-supported
or conventional
prosthesis

⏷

Yes

⏷

Ⓑ Adequate anchorage for routine space closure ⟶ Yes ⟶ Conventional
orthodontics

⏷

No

⏷

Ⓒ Adequate site for implant distal to third molar

Yes   No

⏷   ⏷

Ⓓ Place 7-10 mm implant   Ⓔ Place implant in edentulous
leaving it 1-2 mm above   space as far mesial as possible
the bone level

⏷   ⏷

Uncover in 4 months,   Use implant as anchorage for
place abutment with   mesial movement of molars
anchorage wire or   until optimal pontic width
attach wire directly   is achieved
to implant base

⏷   ⏷

Stabilize sagittal | Implant-Supported Crown |
position of premolar | or Fixed Bridge |
anterior to space

⏷

| Mesial Space Closure |

D. A 7.00 × 3.75 mm retromolar implant is adequate for orthodontic anchorage. A longer implant is unnecessary and may impinge on the inferior alveolar canal. Countersinking of the implant is rarely needed. Protrusion up to 3 mm above the periosteal surface is acceptable because of the thick retromolar soft tissue. After about a 4 month unloaded healing phase, the implant is uncovered, a transcutaneous abutment is installed, or a biocompatible (titanium alloy) wire is attached directly to the endosseous base. An anchorage wire, extending from the abutment, is used to stabilize the sagittal position of the premolar anterior to the edentulous space (Fig. 1). Translation mechanics across the edentulous space results in unidirectional space closure (i.e., molars moving mesially to eliminate the space). It is important to utilize buccal and lingual mechanics (Fig. 2) to avoid periodontal problems that can result from segment rotation and soft tissue pressure on the edentulous ridge.

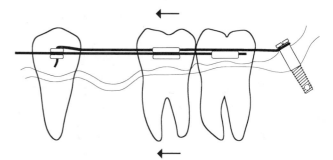

Figure 1. Sagittal view of implant anchored orthodontic mechanism to achieve mesial space closure of second and third molars into a first molar extraction site. (From Roberts WE, Garetto LP, Katona TR. Principles of orthodontic biomechanics: Metabolic and mechanical control mechanisms. In: Carlson DS, Goldstein SA, eds. Bone biodynamics in orthodontic and orthopedic treatment. Ann Arbor: University of Michigan Press, 1992:189.)

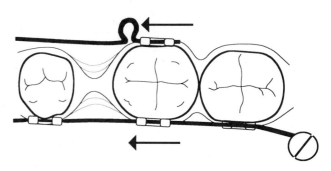

Figure 2. Occlusal view of the implant anchored orthodontic mechanism shown in Figure 1 demonstrates shielding of the periosteal surface to achieve space closure of an atrophic ridge. (From Roberts WE, Garetto LP, Katona TR. Principles of orthodontic biomechanics: Metabolic and mechanical control mechanisms. In: Carlson DS, Goldstein SA, eds. Bone biodynamics in orthodontic and orthopedic treatment. Ann Arbor: University of Michigan Press, 1992:189.)

E. In the absence of an adequate site for an anchorage implant or if there is another limitation, some orthodontic correction to minimize the space is desirable to decrease the mechanical demands on the subsequent bridge. Place the implant in the edentulous space as far mesial as possible. After healing and abutment installation, the implant is used as anchorage for mesial movement of molars. Once an optimal pontic width and opposing occlusion are achieved, there are three options for restoring the residual space: (1) independent implant-supported crown, (2) implant-supported crown tied to a natural tooth to control rotation and mechanical fatigue tendencies, or (3) removing the abutment, covering the implant with soft tissue, and restoring the residual space with a conventional three unit fixed prosthesis. A relatively short span fixed bridge may be superior to an implant-supported prosthesis over the long term. Heavy occlusal loading over a lifetime contributes to fatigue failure of the implant, prosthetic components, and/or supporting bone.

References

Adell R, Lekholm U, Rockler B, Brånemark P-I. A 15-year study of osseointegrated implants in the treatment of the edentulous jaw. Int J Oral Surg 1981; 10:387.

Higuchi KW, Slack JM. The use of titanium fixtures for intraoral anchorage to facilitate orthodontic tooth movement. Int J Oral Maxillofac Implants 1991; 3:338.

Meskin LH, Brown LJ, Burnelle JA, Warren GB. Patterns of tooth loss and accumulated prosthetic treatment potential in U.S. employed adults and seniors, 1985–86. Ger 1988; 4:126.

Roberts WE, Garetto LP, Katona TR. Principles of orthodontic biomechanics: Metabolic and mechanical control mechanisms. In: Carlson DS, Goldstein SA, eds. Bone biodynamics in orthodontic and orthopedic treatment. Ann Arbor: University of Michigan Press, 1992:189.

Roberts WE, Marshall KJ, Mozsary PG. Rigid endosseous implant utilized as anchorage to protract molars and close an atrophic extraction site. Angle Orthod 1990; 60:135.

NONRESTORABLE SPACE IN THE MAXILLA

David B. Clark

Occasionally, patients present with nonrestorable space in the maxillary arch. Generally, this space is insufficient for the placement of a pontic and yet too large to allow space closure through modest overcontouring of proximal contacts. Space problems develop as a result of early tooth loss, congenitally missing teeth, and tooth size anomalies. The permanent first molar is frequently lost to caries or periodontal disease. This often results in considerable mesial drift of the second and third molars while the premolars drift distally. Anteriorly, incisors are frequently lost as a result of trauma. Maxillary lateral incisors are among the teeth most often diminished in size, "peg shaped," or congenitally missing. Unmanaged space frequently leads to undesirable tipping, rotation, and drifting of teeth.

A. The first consideration in management of maxillary anterior space is whether adequate overjet exists to allow for complete space closure. Inadequate overjet necessitates management of the space rather than space closure. A diagnostic set-up should be used to determine the most ideal occlusion.

B. Midline deviations are an important consideration. Once the best occlusion is determined, the specific tooth movements dictate if space should be opened for a pontic or equalized on the mesial and distal surfaces of one or several teeth. Several small interproximal spaces are often easier to restore than a large asymmetric one.

C. Midline deviations and posterior dental symmetry should be considered conjointly when adequate overjet exists for space closure. Unilateral space closure may result in a midline deviation. A diagnostic set-up is indicated to assess the optimum occlusion. Midline deviations toward the space usually worsen with space closure. A midline deviation away from the space may improve with space closure. In all cases a change in posterior symmetry involves consideration of interarch occlusal relationships.

D. The first decision for management of posterior space involves posterior crown tipping. Uprighting molars facilitates oral hygiene, reduces mesial pseudopockets, and allows advantageous remodeling of the alveolar process. A diagnostic set-up helps differentiate treatment options: (1) establishing a space the width of the missing tooth, (2) opening space less than the width of the missing tooth, (3) completing the space closure, or (4) equalizing the space mesially and distally for proximal restoration.

E. Crossbites and/or rotations complicate treatment and may be difficult to retain. Comprehensive treatment is required to correct *skeletal* crossbites. Dental crossbites may be corrected orthodontically. Crossbite and rotation correction is often indicated for preprosthetic alignments.

F. If the space is 1 mm or less and cannot be closed, equalizing space on the mesial and distal for restoration of proximal contacts should be considered. This option may also be viable for spaces greater than 1 mm if indicated by the diagnostic set-up.

G. Treatment options include (1) space closure and retention, (2) reopening of the space for restoration with a fixed or removable partial denture, or (3) equalizing the space on the mesial and distal surfaces and restoring the proximal contacts. In most cases treatment is best performed with fixed appliances. Space closure is usually the most challenging technically and may involve comprehensive treatment. Conversely, opening space can often be accomplished with limited appliances. Alveolar ridge atrophy is unfavorable for space closure.

References

Moyers RE. Handbook of orthodontics. 4th ed. Chicago: Year Book Medical Publishers, 1988:74, 233.
Proffit WR. Contemporary orthodontics. 2nd ed. St Louis: Mosby, 1993:219-224, 553-606.

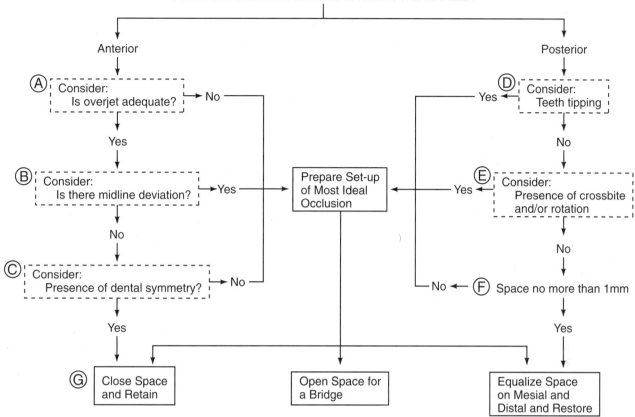

Patient with NONRESTORABLE SPACE IN THE MAXILLA

Anterior

(A) Consider: Is overjet adequate? → No

Yes

(B) Consider: Is there midline deviation? → Yes

No

(C) Consider: Presence of dental symmetry? → No

Yes

Posterior

(D) Consider: Teeth tipping

Yes

No

(E) Consider: Presence of crossbite and/or rotation

Yes

No

(F) Space no more than 1mm → No

Yes

Prepare Set-up of Most Ideal Occlusion

(G) Close Space and Retain

Open Space for a Bridge

Equalize Space on Mesial and Distal and Restore

FLARED MAXILLARY INCISORS

James J. Baldwin
Gordon R. Arbuckle

The esthetic problem of flared and/or spaced maxillary incisors is often a cause of great concern to both adult and adolescent patients. The successful orthodontic correction of this condition requires careful attention to the periodontium and perioral musculature and, most importantly, the determination of the etiology of the flared nature of the teeth. The dentition's position is dictated by the active forces to which it is subjected (e.g., the forces of occlusion, influence of the perioral musculature, abnormal swallowing patterns, and long-term habits [thumb or finger sucking]). The magnification of these effects, superimposed on a dentition losing periodontal support, causes drifting and migration of periodontally involved teeth. The practitioner must carefully evaluate the total patient status and cause of the flaring before attempting to move incisors from a relatively stable position to a less stable one.

A. A comprehensive assessment of the patient's periodontal status is the initial step toward a satisfactory solution. Bleeding on probing is one of the most reliable indicators of inflammation. Inflammatory disease and pocket depths in excess of 3 mm require evaluation and treatment prior to tooth movement. Modest recession (<2 mm) does not contraindicate orthodontic movement, but greater recession in the presence of minimal attached gingiva requires careful evaluation. Areas with less than 2 mm of keratinized gingiva should be considered a potential problem and managed before orthodontic therapy is initiated. A tooth with less than 1 mm of attached gingiva is considered a candidate for grafting. Radiographic evidence of significant alveolar bone defects requires complete evaluation and treatment prior to tooth movement. A tooth with substantial bone loss requires fixed appliances and carefully controlled forces if the teeth are to be repositioned in a controlled fashion.

B. If a pernicious habit is the etiology of flared and spaced incisors, the elimination of the habit is essential to resolving the problem. Altering an improper swallowing pattern or convincing an adolescent to give up a thumb habit is a therapeutic challenge, but it is necessary if a stable result is to be obtained.

C. A "trapped" lower lip is a common pernicious habit. If it is in a constant lingual position to the maxillary incisors, it causes or at least contributes to the flared nature of the dentition. Reversal of this muscular imbalance by initiating lip posture exercises that direct forces from the labial aspect of the dentition not only aids in the correction of the problem but insures the long-term stability of the result.

D. Excessive overjet can have a dental anatomic etiology. The tooth mass of the maxillary and mandibular six anterior teeth does not always dictate an ideal overjet and overbite relationship when the buccal segments are in Class I occlusion. Excessive maxillary tooth mass could dictate excessive overjet unless interproximal reduction is used to eliminate the excess tooth mass. In a similar fashion, malformed teeth such as pegged or missing lateral incisors require a treatment plan that leaves adequate space for esthetic restorations or replacements. To properly assess such problems, a prosthodontic evaluation is necessary (i.e., determination of the nature and size of the final restorations).

E. Simple tipping of maxillary incisors with a removable appliance to close and retract anterior teeth is rarely a viable option. Excessive overbite due to extruded mandibular incisors often accompanies flared maxillary anterior teeth. Removable appliances complicate the problem further because they tend to extrude anterior teeth as they are retracted. Fixed appliances to manage intrusion and/or control axial inclination are usually required. The diagnostic skills necessary to produce an excellent result with partial treatment are more demanding than comprehensive care with full appliances.

F. The stability of completed treatment is a function of the diagnosis. Pernicious habits that persist cause the original malocclusion to return once the retainers are removed because the etiologic factor has not been addressed. If the final treatment position of the tooth is in a balanced position with regard to function and oral-facial musculature, a reasonable period of retention (about 6 months) with a removable appliance should maintain the result. A bonded (fixed) lingual retainer may be required to preserve the closure of a long-standing diastema.

References

Hall WB: Decision making in periodontology. Philadelphia: BC Decker, 1988.

Moyers RE. Handbook of orthodontics. 4th ed. Chicago: Yearbook Medical Publishers, 1988.

Profitt WR. Contemporary orthodontics. 2nd ed. St Louis: Mosby, 1993:576-581.

Patient with FLARED MAXILLARY INCISORS

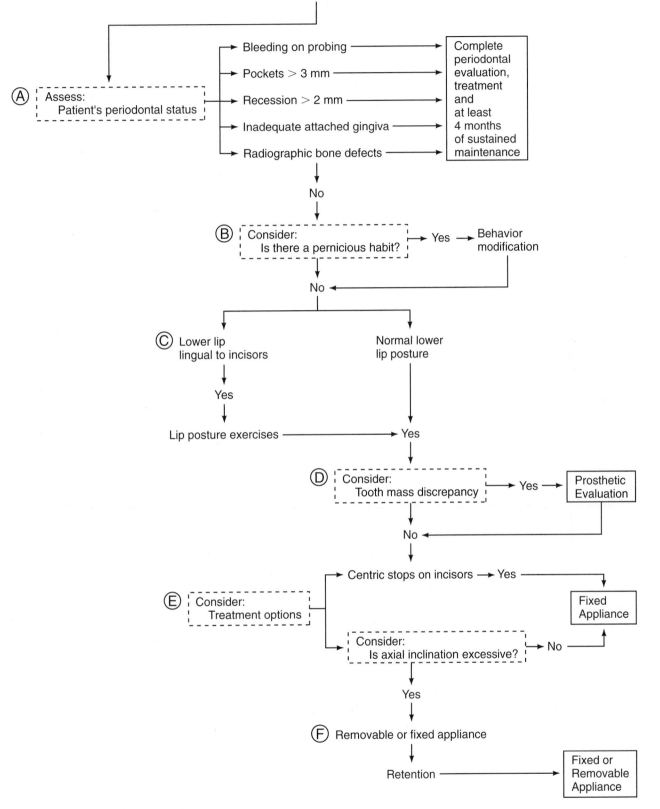

A Assess:
Patient's periodontal status

Bleeding on probing

Pockets > 3 mm

Recession > 2 mm

Inadequate attached gingiva

Radiographic bone defects

Complete periodontal evaluation, treatment and at least 4 months of sustained maintenance

No

B Consider:
Is there a pernicious habit? → Yes → Behavior modification

No

C Lower lip lingual to incisors

Normal lower lip posture

Yes

Lip posture exercises → Yes

D Consider:
Tooth mass discrepancy → Yes → Prosthetic Evaluation

No

E Consider:
Treatment options

Centric stops on incisors → Yes

Fixed Appliance

Consider:
Is axial inclination excessive? → No

Yes

F Removable or fixed appliance

Retention → Fixed or Removable Appliance

153

ORTHODONTIC CROWN LENGTHENING OF A FRACTURED TOOTH

William F. Hohlt

Acute, iatrogenic trauma frequently fractures a natural tooth so that the remaining root structure is partially or completely below crestal alveolar bone. Restorations requiring subcrestal finishing lines have been accomplished by using invasive flap procedures with subsequent removal of crestal alveolar bone below the intended finishing line. When conditions are acceptable, an alternative approach is to orthodontically extrude the tooth to the point where the finish line is exposed. This also allows for longer crown preparations to prevent retentive failure and redevelopment of a 2 mm biological width of attached gingiva. Restorative materials that impinge on the biological width stimulate inflammation and irreversible damage in the form of periodontal pocket formation.

A. How far to erupt a tooth root relates to its *final use*. For single crown restorations without a post and core, the projected crown length should not exceed the root length in bone (Figs. 1 and 2). If a post and core restoration is planned, the projected crown length should equal the post length inserted into the tooth root. It is safe to project crown-to-root ratios of 1:1.5; however, Dykema et al. state that crown:root ratios as small as 1:1 can be utilized when such circumstances prevail.

Oppenheim reported in 1940 that artificially elongated teeth stimulated the entire alveolar process to follow in the direction of eruption. He also observed that light eruptive forces promoted formation of crestal osteoid while strong eruptive forces caused supracrestal fiber tearing with no associated osteoid formation.

Supracrestal fiberotomy can be designed to prevent crestal bone development in areas where crestal bone and periodontium are healthy and stimulate development in areas adjacent to healthy gingivae with crestal bone defects. If a tooth is fractured at the level of crestal bone involving 360 degrees of root surface, supracrestal fiberotomy is advised to forcibly erupt the fractured root without stimulating crestal bone formation. If there is an oblique root fracture where part of the root is fractured below the crestal bone, a supracrestal fiberotomy should be performed on the root area that has normal attachment until the oblique fractured root surface has erupted to the level of crestal bone, at which time 360 degree weekly crestal fiberotomies should be performed. In cases involving oblique fractures it is necessary to equilibrate the erupting fragment if occlusal trauma is noted from the opposing occlusion. By severing the supracrestal fibers, the tooth root will quickly (in 3 to 4 weeks) extrude from the bone. *Archwire segments should be activated to ideal projected needs rather than be overactivated when supracrestal fiberotomies are performed.* Under this circumstance there is little resistance to tooth movement and the tooth can be pulled out of its periodontal support.

B. In cases where the tooth needing extrusion has had previous endodontic treatment, a small fabricated eyelet can be inserted in the prepared pulp canal and cemented in place with Durelon. The eyelet is constructed from 0.020 inch stainless steel wire in such a way as to have a corkscrew appearance. Alternatively, small cross members welded onto the wire also provide resistance from dislodgment. In cases where there is either no enamel to bond an appliance or no pulp canal to insert an eyelet, attachment is improvised using a custom-pinched band or temporary casting.

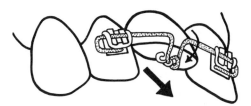

Figure 1. Mechanics to extrude an incisor along its long axis.

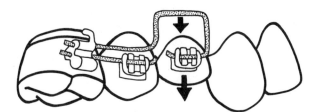

Figure 2. Premolar extrusion to achieve a 1:1 crown:root ratio.

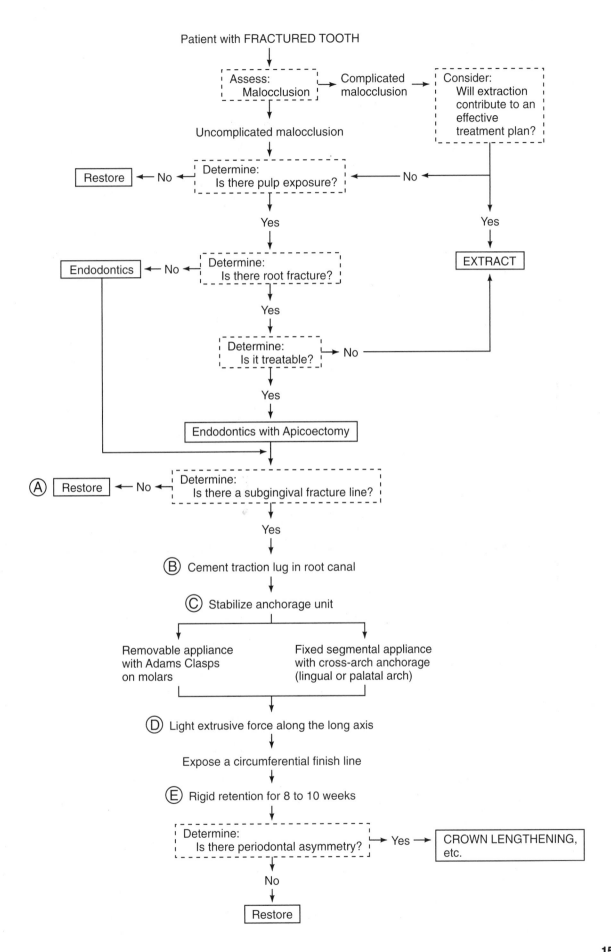

Patient with FRACTURED TOOTH

Assess: Malocclusion → Complicated malocclusion → Consider: Will extraction contribute to an effective treatment plan?

Uncomplicated malocclusion

Restore ← No ← Determine: Is there pulp exposure? ← No ←

Yes

Endodontics ← No ← Determine: Is there root fracture?

Yes

Determine: Is it treatable? → No →

Yes

EXTRACT

Endodontics with Apicoectomy

(A) Restore ← No ← Determine: Is there a subgingival fracture line?

Yes

(B) Cement traction lug in root canal

(C) Stabilize anchorage unit

Removable appliance with Adams Clasps on molars

Fixed segmental appliance with cross-arch anchorage (lingual or palatal arch)

(D) Light extrusive force along the long axis

Expose a circumferential finish line

(E) Rigid retention for 8 to 10 weeks

Determine: Is there periodontal asymmetry? → Yes → CROWN LENGTHENING, etc.

No

Restore

C. A simple definition of anchorage is described by Proffit as "resistance to unwanted tooth movement". For purposes of root lengthening it must be remembered that extrusive movement occurs more quickly than intrusive movement; nevertheless, sound anchorage requirements must be observed to eliminate undesirable side effects. A single tooth root can be extruded using adjacent anchorage units with two to three times the reactive tooth root's surface area. For example, two premolars and a canine may serve as anchorage against an extrusive attempt on a first molar. A central incisor is easily extruded using adjacent central and lateral incisors as anchor units.

D. Methods of tooth extrusion may be simple, such as tying elastic thread between a tooth root and an anchor unit, or they may involve more sophisticated force systems. The method described requires very little reactivation. It takes advantage of the torsion and bending properties of wires to extrude teeth. Figure 3 demonstrates eruption of tooth 31 using teeth 30, 29, and 28 as anchorage units. A 0.014 inch round stainless steel wire segment is fabricated so that the terminal segment of wire engages the bracket of tooth 28 by doubling back superior to the bracket wing. This doubled-back wire prevents the segment from rolling as the wire's other end is twisted and tied to the attachment of tooth 31. As the energy in the spring wire dissipates, the reactive end extrudes the molar root for the first 3 to 4 mm of the arc. It is wise to limit the activation of the wire to no more than 4 mm in case the patient fails to return for adjustment 3 to 4 weeks later. Greater activation could result in excessive extrusion and buccal tipping.

The anchorage units are splinted together with a stiff rectangular wire, 0.018 × 0.025 inch (0.018 inch bracket slot) while the 0.014 inch erupting wire is tied in piggyback fashion to the heavier stabilizing segment. Figure 1 demonstrates a similar design for a central incisor where once again the 0.014 inch segment doubles back incisal to the bracket wings on teeth 7 and 10, thus resisting rotation. Figure 2 demonstrates a more common approach to premolar root extrusion where a rectangular loop configuration provides the eruptive force. In this case the anchorage units have again been splinted together with a heavy rectangular arch wire. The active arch wire is attached to an auxiliary bracket tube on the first molar.

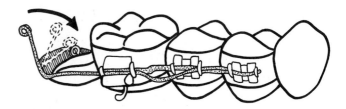

Figure 3. Demonstration of how tooth extrudes for first 3 to 4 degrees of arc. Note how erupting wire wraps back around occlusal of bracket wing on first premolar, providing resistance to torsion.

E. Once the tooth has erupted satisfactorily, a brief period of stabilization is needed. Activation should be discontinued and the tooth held in its new position for approximately 8 to 10 weeks. Stabilization can be effected using either a passive wire or the deactivated erupting spring.

References

Dykema RW. Johnson's modern practice in fixed prosthodontics. 4th ed. Philadelphia: WB Saunders, 1986:10.

Gargiulo AW, Wentz FM, Orban B. Dimensions of the dentogingival junction in humans. J Periodont 1961; 32:261.

Oppenheim A. Artificial elongation of the teeth. Am J Orthod Oral Surg 1940; 26:931.

Parma-Benfenati S, Fugazzotto PA, Ruben MP. The effect of restorative margins on the postsurgical development and nature of the periodontium. Part 1. Int J Periodont Restor Dent 1985; 5(6):31.

Polson A, Caton J, Polson AP, et al. Periodontal response after tooth movement into infrabony defects. J Periodont 1984; 55(4):197.

Pontoriero R, Celenza F, Ricci G, et al. Rapid extrusion with fiber resection: A combined orthodontic periodontic treatment modality. Int J Periodont Restor Dent 1987; 7(5):31.

Proffit WR. Contemporary orthodontics. 2nd ed. St Louis: Mosby, 1993:260.

Simon JHS, Kelly WH, Gordon DG, et al. Extrusion of endodontically treated teeth. J Am Dent Assoc 1978; 97:17.

ORTHODONTICS AND PURE MUCOGINGIVAL PROBLEMS IN THE TRANSITIONAL DENTITION

Neal Murphy

A. A distinction must be made between the growing and the nongrowing patient when evaluating the clinical significance of mucogingival problems for planning orthodontic treatment. Frank skeletal dysplasia (jaw malalignment) can exacerbate the pernicious effects of pure mucogingival orthodontic problems (i.e., a developing deep bite introduces the effects of direct gingival impingement by food and incisor contact on preexisting inadequate attached gingiva).

B. Development of mucogingival problems can be anticipated in the primary dentition. If generalized spacing is evident throughout the anterior sextants, the chance of crowding is minimal. Interproximal contact of the primary teeth without crowding (arch length deficiency) may portend anterior crowding, and crowded primary teeth will evolve into a crowded permanent dentition.

C. Extraction of a deciduous tooth when the succedaneous tooth demonstrates 75% or more root formation can accelerate the permanent tooth eruption. Less than a 75% root formation on a succedaneous tooth suggests a delayed eruption of the permanent tooth if the primary mate is extracted. When 75% of the root is formed and the eruption trajectory leads to alveolar mucosa, the primary tooth should be extracted to allow the permanent tooth to erupt into gingiva.

D. The mixed dentition, particularly at the transition stage, marks a critical opportunity to ameliorate or preempt a developing malocclusion. When patient cooperation is optimal functional appliances can produce marked changes at this time. Indolent mucogingival pathoses may develop into clinical entities.

E. Judicious serial extraction allows developing crowding in the mandibular anterior sextant to realign distally, relieving stress on the mandibular anterior attached gingiva.

F. Nonextraction therapy may consist of movement of mandibular teeth anteriorly or interproximal enamel reduction (stripping) to gain space for the realignment of teeth. Prophylactic or therapeutic gingival augmentation is difficult if an overbite (vertical overlap of the anterior teeth) impinges on the mandibular anterior gingival margin.

G. Overbite is not an encumbering factor if sufficient overjet (horizontal overlap of the anterior teeth) is sufficient to allow the surgeon adequate room to operate and place protective periodontal surgical dressing. Generally, 2 mm is sufficient overjet to preclude incisor impingement on the mandibular surgical site.

   The secondary dentition in the growing patient presents greater necessity for extraction therapy in the repositioning of lower incisors lingually, away from a stressed labial attached gingiva. If extraction therapy is employed to reduce labial protrusion, additional salutary effects are often seen as the thin attached gingiva becomes thicker and more resistant to insult.

References

Coatoam GW, Behrents RG, Bissada NF. The width of traumatized gingiva during orthodontic treatment: Its significance and impact on periodontal status. J Peridontol 1981; 52:307.

Dorfman HS. Mucogingival changes resulting from mandibular incisor tooth movement. Am J Orthod 1978; 74:286.

Hall WB. Pure mucogingival problems. Berlin: Quintessence Publishing, 1989:44, 68, 178.

Maynard JG, Ochsenbein C. Mucogingival problems, prevalence and therapy in children. J. Periodontol 1975; 46:543.

Proceedings of World Workshop in Clinical Periodontics. Chicago: American Academy of Periodontology, 1989.

Patient for ORTHODONTICS WITH MANDIBULAR INCISOR LACKING ATTACHED GINGIVA

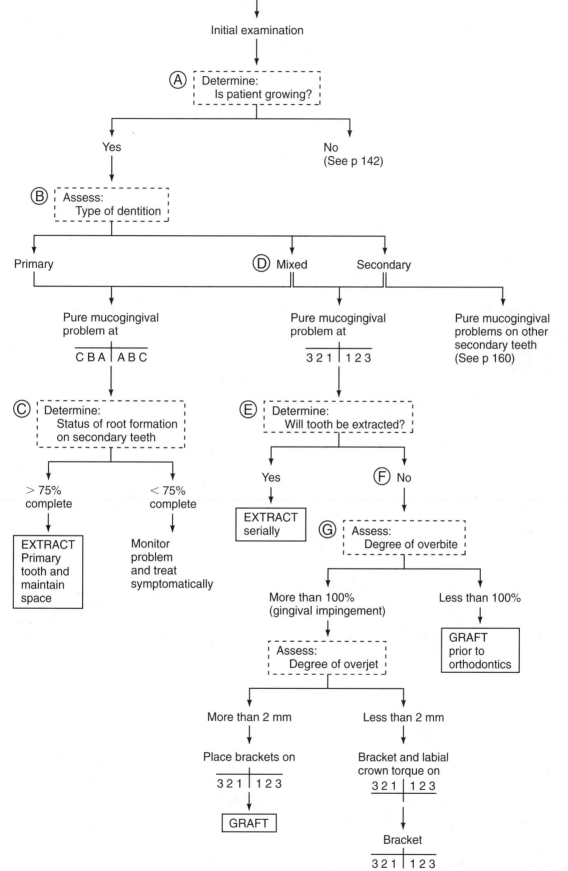

PURE MUCOGINGIVAL PROBLEMS IN ADULT ORTHODONTIC CASES

Neal Murphy

A. Extraction of teeth to eliminate crowding keeps the remaining teeth within the confines of the existing alveolar bone and gingiva. If nonextraction techniques of space gaining are employed (except for interproximal enamel reduction), stress on the dentogingival unit follows, presenting a potential for bony dehiscence and gingival recession. This occurs if the osteoblastic activity of fibroplasia does not compensate by accommodating the new tooth position space. If less than 1 mm of attached gingiva is present, grafting should precede tooth movement.

B. Generally, a slower expansion of the dental arch transversely or anteriorly allows the attachment apparatus sufficient time to accommodate the teeth in their new positions. This occurs if (1) the new position lies within the phenotypical potential of the attached gingiva and alveoli, and (2) infection is controlled. If active recession occurs, however, grafting is needed.

C. Rapid expansion generally results in more tooth movement than scalable expansion, greater tipping movement of the teeth, and greater relapse potential, in addition to the increase in dehiscence potential.

D. If esthetic demands dictate that roots be covered with gingiva, the histologic attachment to the treated tooth surface may be epithelial. The only histologic continuity between soft tissue and root is hemidesmosomal with a thin coating of mucopolysaccharides. The possibility of new connective tissue attachment to new cementum using Sharpey's fibers is conjectural; thus, if no esthetic imperative dictates root coverage, a submarginal free gingival graft should be employed to increase the attached gingiva.

E. One of the limitations of root coverage in providing a predictable new attachment is that the adjacent donor site does not present sufficient dense fibrous connective tissue to employ a pedicle grafting technique. In such a case, a free connective tissue graft must be used in conjunction with a marsupialized adjacent mucosa.

F. If interproximal enamel reduction or tooth extraction gains sufficient room to treat arch length deficiency, attached gingiva can prove inadequate to resist the destructive forces of bacterial infection and mechanical orthodontic tooth movement.

Where the existing attached gingiva is less than 1 mm, close monitoring by the dentist and patient should meet the demands of both professional and legal imperatives. The potential for precipitous gingival dehiscence in an area of adequate attached gingiva (greater than 1 mm) are rare enough to justify monitoring by the dentist and the orthodontist during professional visits (usually every 4 to 6 weeks).

References

Carranza FA. Clinical periodontology. 7th ed. Philadelphia: WB Saunders, 1990:875.

Corn H. Reconstructive mucogingival surgery. In: Goldman HM, Cohen DW, eds. Periodontal therapy. 6th ed. St Louis: Mosby, 1980:795.

Hall WB. Pure mucogingival problems. Berlin: Quintessence Publishing, 1984.

Hall WB. Gingival augmentation/mucogingival surgery. In: World Workshop in Clinical Periodontics. Chicago: American Academy of Periodontology, 1989:VII-1.

Schluger S, Yuodelis R, Page RC, Johnson RH. Periodontal disease. 2nd ed. Philadelphia: Lea & Febiger, 1990:458.

Adult orthodontic patient with LACK OF ATTACHED GINGIVA ON POSTERIOR TEETH

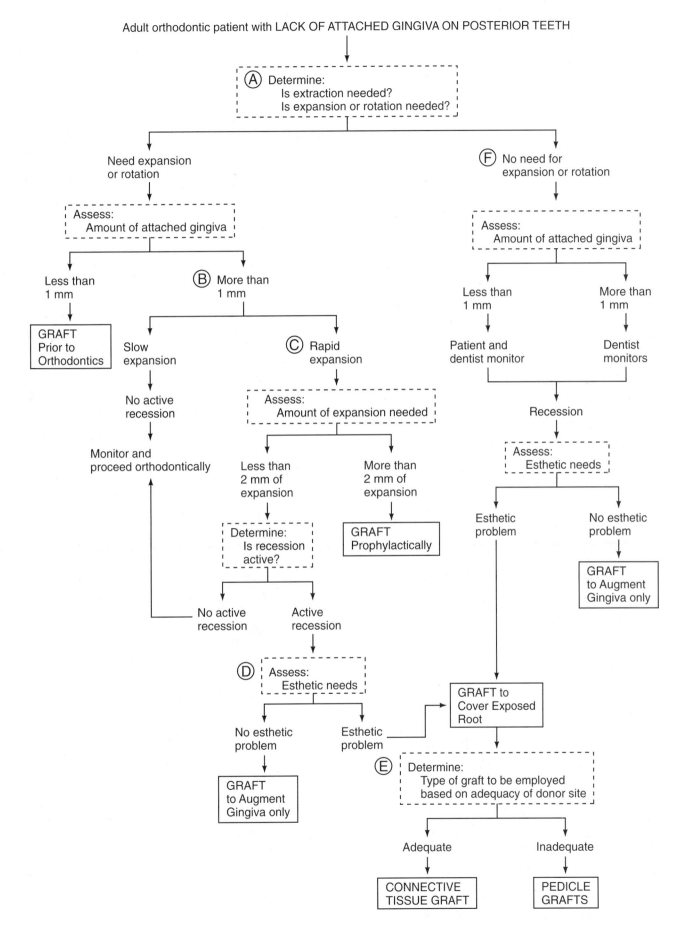

161

PROSTHODONTICS

Eugene E. LaBarre, Editor

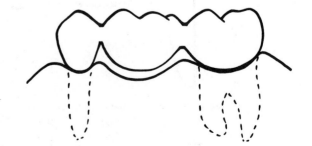

FIXED PARTIAL DENTURE VERSUS REMOVABLE PARTIAL DENTURE

Eugene E. LaBarre

As a general rule, fixed tooth replacement is preferred over removable restorations because of greater patient convenience and acceptance. On the other hand, a removable partial denture (RPD) can be designed for virtually every partially edentulous patient; the fixed partial denture (FPD) has biomechanical limits that restrict its application (Fig. 1). In addition, financial considerations may be compelling; a removable prosthesis may be chosen in a case where a fixed restoration is biologically feasible but too expensive for the patient.

A. A single missing tooth is best replaced by a conventional FPD or implant. If a lateral or small central incisor is absent and the occlusal stresses are not traumatic, it can be replaced by a cantilever pontic supported by a canine or central incisor. Although the simple FPD procedure is predictable and successful, the presence of virgin abutment teeth argues for an adhesive FPD or a single tooth implant.

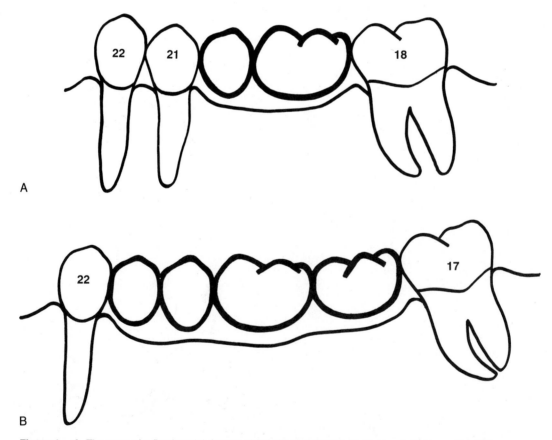

Figure 1. A, The span of a fixed partial denture should be restricted to posterior edentulous areas of three teeth or less. **B,** A removable partial denture can be designed to restore any edentulous space but is particularly useful for long spans involving three or more posterior teeth.

Patient who is PARTIALLY EDENTULOUS FOR WHOM IMPLANT TREATMENT HAS BEEN RULED OUT

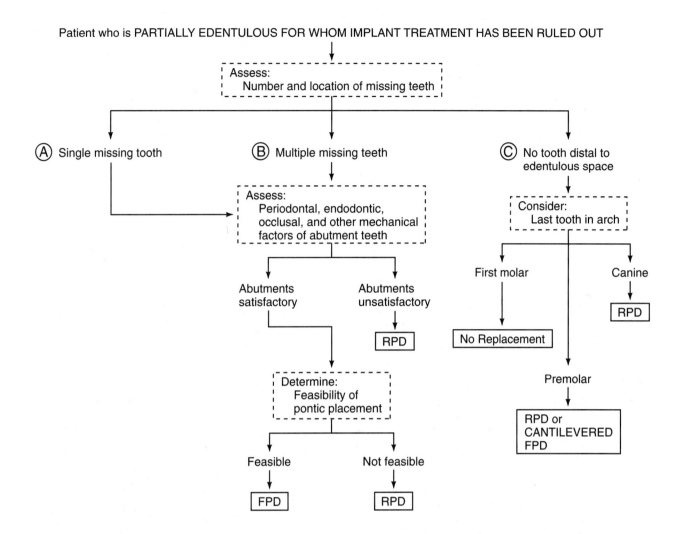

B. A number of conditions should be met before a FPD is planned to replace multiple missing teeth. Mechanical considerations require a complex FPD to be supported by an adequate number of sound abutments (roughly equal to the teeth being replaced) of sufficient occlusogingival length to retain the restoration with controlled occlusal forces. The need for periodontal and endodontic health in abutments is the same for fixed and removable restorations, but a complex FPD is much more of a commitment for a patient than its removable counterpart and has no reversibility or convertibility. An ailing FPD abutment can condemn the entire restoration.

C. In situations where all posterior teeth are missing, the distal extension RPD is the treatment of choice. If premolars are present and occlusion does not require replacement of both first and second molars, a

cantilevered FPD utilizing multiple abutments to support an undersized pontic posteriorly may be acceptable. Patients with intact dentitions posteriorly to the first molar have adequate occlusal function as do many patients with second premolar occlusion.

References

McDermott IG, Grasso JE. Removable partial overdentures. Dent Clin North Am 1990; 34:611.

Renner RP, Boucher LJ. Removable partial dentures. Chicago: Quintessence Publishing, 1987:151.

Shillingburg HT, Hobo S, Whitsett LD. Fundamentals of fixed prosthodontics. 2nd ed. Chicago: Quintessence Publishing, 1981:17.

Stockstill JW, Bowley JF, Attanasio R. Clinical decision analysis in fixed prosthodontics. Dent Clin North Am 1992; 36:569.

PROSTHODONTIC IMPLICATIONS OF A HOPELESS TOOTH

Eugene E. LaBarre

A common clinical situation is that of a single problem tooth in an otherwise intact dental arch. The problem may be the result of chronic inflammatory processes or trauma. If the most predictable and logical treatment for the tooth is extraction, the tooth is considered hopeless.

A. Occasionally, a patient with a hopeless tooth insists that the tooth be salvaged rather than extracted. Such a request must be balanced by the dentist's professional judgment regarding the feasibility of heroic treatment. To help the patient make a well-informed decision, the cause of the problem must be diagnosed and explained.

B. The majority of isolated hopeless teeth have problems that are readily identified: severe periodontitis, failing endodontics, failing root integrity owing to cracks or resorption, and severe fracture of coronal tooth structure (Fig. 1). All of these conditions are difficult and expensive to treat, and the short-term prognosis remains uncertain. The dentist must have a frank discussion with the patient, so that the costs and the potential for failure are fully disclosed.

C. If the patient has no interest in pursuing heroic treatment or if salvage of the tooth is attempted and fails, the tooth is extracted. Short-term replacement possibilities include the stayplate or provisional fixed partial denture (FPD). Definitive replacement therapies are highly predictable: single tooth implant, FPD, or removable partial denture (RPD).

D. If the patient has opted for heroic treatment and the dental problem has been stabilized by preliminary therapy, restoration of the tooth itself is the most desirable treatment. With a mobile tooth, some form of reversibility is desirable in the splint or FPD so that future problems with the tooth can be managed without sacrifice of the restoration. Telescopic restorations are mentioned, because the possibility exists for removing the restorations from cemented copings. However, the patient must understand that redoing prosthodontic restorations is always a possibility when future events are difficult to predict. Compliance with regular recall is essential for maintenance of a single hopeless tooth.

References

Cohen S, Burns RC. Pathways of the pulp. 5th ed. St Louis: Mosby—Year Book, 1991:738.

Geurtsen W. The cracked-tooth syndrome: Clinical features and case reports. Int J Periodont Restor Dent 1992; 12:395.

Laney WR, Tolman DE. Tissue integration in oral, orthopedic, and maxillofacial reconstruction. Chicago: Quintessence Publishing, 1990:203.

Lindhe J. Textbook of clinical periodontology. Philadelphia: WB Saunders, 1983:501.

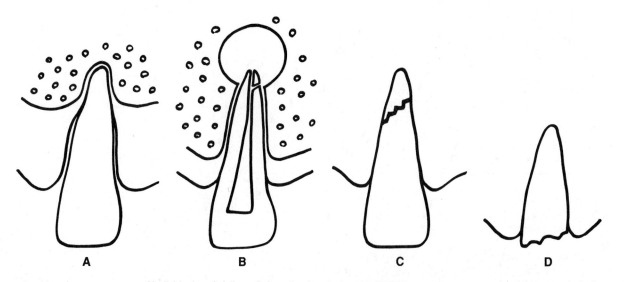

Figure 1. Most frequent causes of individual tooth failure. **A,** Localized periodontitis. **B,** Failing endodontic seal. **C,** Root fracture. **D,** Coronal destruction.

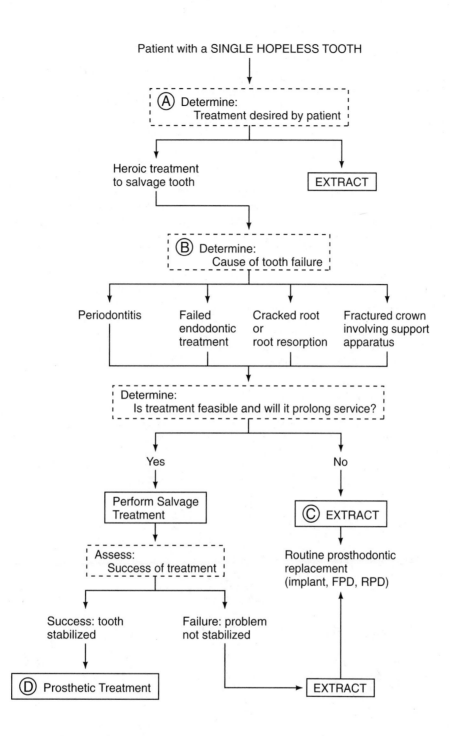

Patient with a SINGLE HOPELESS TOOTH

A Determine:
Treatment desired by patient

Heroic treatment to salvage tooth

EXTRACT

B Determine:
Cause of tooth failure

Periodontitis

Failed endodontic treatment

Cracked root or root resorption

Fractured crown involving support apparatus

Determine:
Is treatment feasible and will it prolong service?

Yes

No

Perform Salvage Treatment

C EXTRACT

Assess:
Success of treatment

Routine prosthodontic replacement (implant, FPD, RPD)

Success: tooth stabilized

Failure: problem not stabilized

D Prosthetic Treatment

EXTRACT

PROSTHODONTIC ASPECTS OF THE EXTENSIVELY DAMAGED DENTITION

Eugene E. LaBarre

A patient with extensively damaged dentition suffers from generalized advanced dental pathology, including periodontitis, caries, or occlusal trauma. The patient may have neglected his dental health, or, even if regular treatment has been received, the patient's problems may have become so advanced that treatment is no longer effective or predictable. The "downhill" mouth has been described extensively, including a remarkable study by Nyman and Lindhe describing the long-term periodontal and prosthodontic rehabilitation in these patients. The success and predictability of endosseous dental implants have added another dimension to the treatment of truly hopeless cases. Planning and executing the rehabilitation that best suits the individual patient are great challenges in dentistry.

A. The examination and diagnosis must be thorough. In particular, the success or failure of previous and prospective treatment must be determined. The patient must demonstrate a willingness and determination to participate in the treatment before any extensive rehabilitation is attempted. If there is any question about this important phase of treatment, it may be desirable to stabilize the dental pathology with interim restorations until satisfactory results are demonstrated. If the interim phase of treatment is a failure, it is possible to move on to extractions and removable prostheses without major sacrifice of time and energy.

B. Maintenance treatment may be effective in slowing or arresting early phases of pathology (e.g., before tooth mobility and migration have occurred). Generally, when multiple teeth are missing or when the mouth is in an advanced state of disrepair, maintenance is of questionable value.

C. The salvage of teeth by extensive periodontal, endodontic, and prosthetic treatment has been shown to stabilize dental health in patients who learn effective home care regimens. However, many patients are not capable of such outstanding hygiene year after year. The telescopic prosthesis was developed to permit fixed splinting and tooth replacement with a restoration that could be removed from individual copings for maintenance and repair. However, any fixed prosthesis placed over teeth with guarded prognoses must be regarded as heroic, high risk treatment.

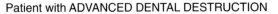

Patient with ADVANCED DENTAL DESTRUCTION

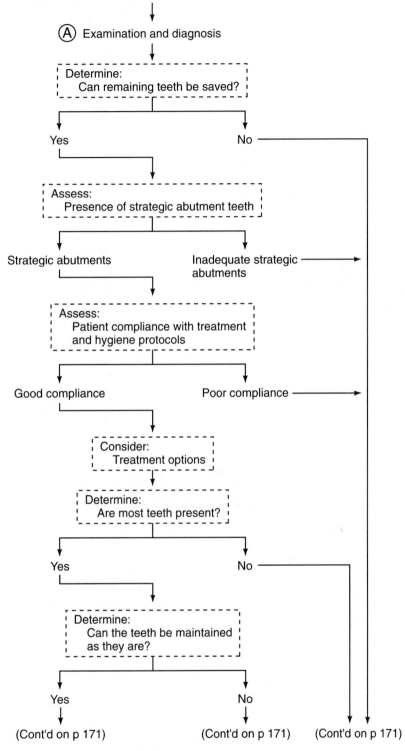

Ⓐ Examination and diagnosis

Determine:
  Can remaining teeth be saved?

Yes   No

Assess:
  Presence of strategic abutment teeth

Strategic abutments   Inadequate strategic
                             abutments

Assess:
  Patient compliance with treatment
  and hygiene protocols

Good compliance   Poor compliance

Consider:
  Treatment options

Determine:
  Are most teeth present?

Yes   No

Determine:
  Can the teeth be maintained
  as they are?

Yes   No

(Cont'd on p 171)   (Cont'd on p 171)   (Cont'd on p 171)

D. A common treatment involves salvaging strategic abutments for a prosthesis and extracting noncritical or problematic teeth. The approach has the advantages of simplifying treatment and maintenance, while providing dental support for the restoration. Strategic teeth are well-supported canines and molars. Minimally, a fixed partial denture (FPD) or tooth-supported removable partial denture (RPD) requires four abutments. A distal extension RPD requires two abutments (Fig. 1).

E. Full mouth extraction is the most drastic treatment in terms of tooth loss but also the most predictable in eliminating dental pathology. The complete denture, particularly in the mandible, can be a very poor substitute for natural teeth. Fortunately, implants can provide anchorage for overdentures to make these restorations highly successful.

References

Lindhe J. Textbook of clinical periodontology. Philadelphia: WB Saunders, 1983:309, 451.

Nyman S, Lindhe J. A longitudinal study of combined periodontal and prosthetic treatment of patients with advanced periodontal disease. J Periodont 1979; 50:163.

Renner RP, Boucher LJ. Removable partial dentures. Chicago: Quintessence Publishing, 1987:151.

Yalisove IL, Dietz JB. Telescopic prosthetic therapy. Philadelphia: GF Stickley, 1977:7.

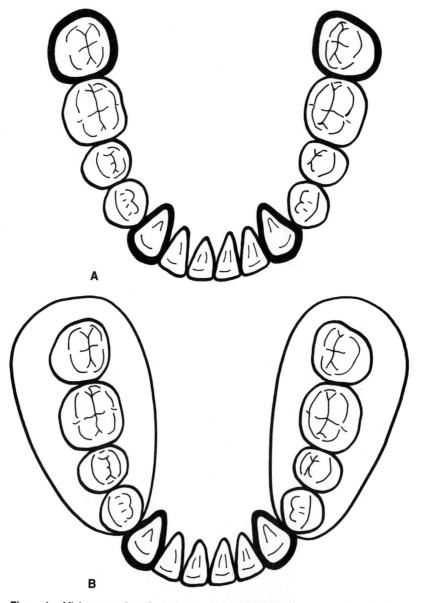

Figure 1. Minimum number of strategic abutments for **(A)** tooth-supported prosthesis—two lateroanterior abutments (canines or premolars) and two posterior abutments (molars); and **(B)** distal extension RPD—two lateroanterior abutments (canines or premolars).

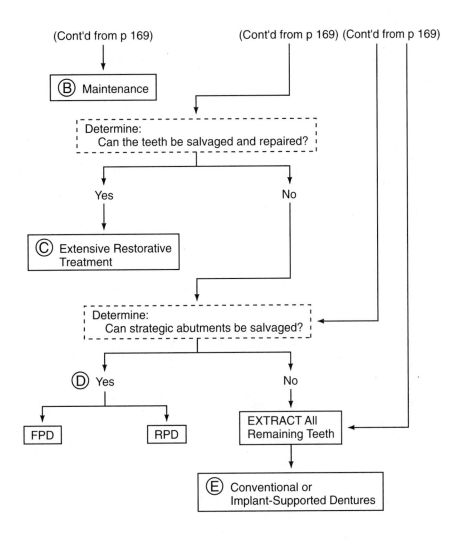

SELECTING INDIVIDUAL TOOTH RESTORATIONS

Chi Tran

Although most dentists would agree that conserving intact tooth structure is as important as restoring the tooth, the PFM crown is the most common cemented restoration. Conservative cast restorations are not as prevalent as in the past because of patients' esthetic demands and time constraints in modern dental practice. Nevertheless, there are functional as well as esthetic criteria for restoring teeth, which determine the type of restoration required.

A. Restorative dentistry in the visible part of the mouth is concerned mainly with tooth-colored restorations. A main objective is to make the restoration inconspicuous to the patient. Porcelain inlays and onlays can reinforce posterior teeth with moderate lesions. The PFM crown restores severely damaged teeth and has broad application in reconstruction of occlusion and esthetics.

B. For posterior teeth that are not prominently visible, restoration of function is the main objective. Partial veneer gold crowns are conservative and offer unparalleled clinical service. Full veneer crowns are required for teeth with short axial walls or for severely damaged teeth. Amalgam and cast gold also have wear properties similar to tooth structure.

C. Because cast restorations are indicated for fixed partial dentures (FPD), retention becomes a more important factor. Partial veneer retainers may be used for simple FPDs, but full coverage is generally recommended because of increased functional demand. Retainers of similar retentive capacity are used to reduce the incidence of partial loosening.

References

Shillingburg HT, Hobo S, Whitsett LD. Fundamentals of fixed prosthodontics. 2nd ed. Chicago: Quintessence Publishing, 1981.

Wall GJ, Cipra DL. Is the metal-ceramic crown always the restoration of choice? Dent Clin North Am 1992; 36:765.

Patient with CARIES or UNSERVICEABLE RESTORATIONS

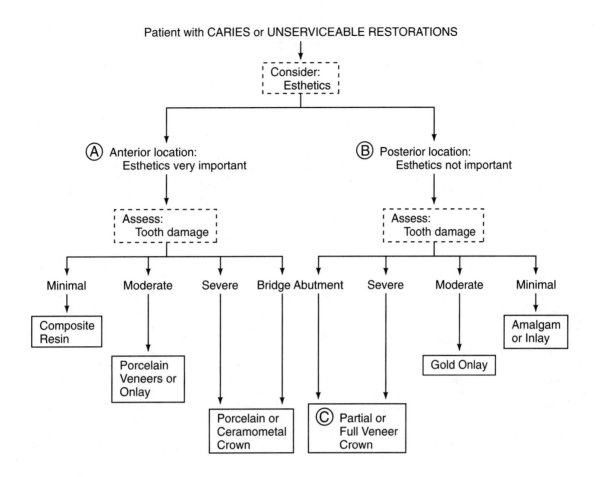

SELECTING FIXED PROSTHODONTIC PROCEDURES

Casimir Leknius

In the present era of rapidly developing alternative prosthodontic techniques, it is useful to review the indications for fixed prosthodontics. These procedures—including individual cast gold or PFM crowns, splinted cast restorations, or fixed partial dentures—constitute the bulk of fixed prosthodontic practice.

A. The most obvious indication for crowns is to restore damaged teeth. Specific guidelines, such as isthmus width of existing intracoronal restorations exceeding certain intercuspal dimensions and/or missing cusps, have been suggested. Generally, it is advisable to restore any tooth weakened by existing restoration or caries where a significant risk of breakage exists. Published diagnostic criteria and indices are useful.

B. Occlusal wear and missing teeth are often associated with severely compromised occlusal schemes, such as an exaggerated or reverse curve of Spee. This usually comes about as a result of extrusion following the extraction of antagonist teeth. Often it is further complicated by prostheses placed in a conformative manner without correction of the occlusal plane. These cases must be carefully analyzed prior to restoration and frequently require the disciplines of endodontics, orthodontics, and surgery for block resections and periodontics for crown lengthening before a predictably successful prosthesis can be placed. It is not prudent to perpetuate malocclusions or iatrogenic occlusal schemes simply because it is an expedient way to replace missing teeth.

It is desirable to match occlusal wear factors in the selection of restorative materials in such cases. PFM restorations have the potential for esthetic match or improvement of the natural teeth, but the increased hardness of porcelain compared with enamel makes this a destructive material choice in areas subjected to heavy parafunction. Composite resins have not yet demonstrated adequate wear resistance to be considered as an esthetic veneer for cast restorations in the posterior quadrants. At the present time, only cast gold alloys and amalgam have wear properties similar to natural tooth structure.

C. Replacement of missing teeth utilizing fixed prosthodontic procedures is a predictable procedure. The possibility of replacing teeth with implants should also be explored (see pp 208 and 210). Fixed partial dentures increase the occlusal load on abutment teeth, necessitating careful diagnostic review of bone support, mobility, crown length, edentulous span, and other factors related to restoration, durability, and strength. Ante's Law, which suggests that root surface area of abutments should equal that of the teeth being replaced, is a good general guideline but is successfully violated on a routine basis in clinical practice. The classic argument against Ante's Law is exemplified by the canine-supported FPD, which replaces four incisors. Individual experience, rather than precise application of rules or guidelines, determines that this is an appropriate restoration for one patient and not for another.

D. Splinting with cast restorations for periodontal or orthodontic stability is another routine application of fixed prosthodontic technology (see p 188). The two main issues to be considered in splinting are whether it is physically possible to splint (in terms of alignment, number of teeth, cost) and whether the teeth are worth the extraordinary effort and difficulty in maintenance of splinting. If there is a possibility of implant placement, heroic restoration of marginal teeth is more difficult to defend now than in the past. Additionally, splinting reduces proprioception and reduces the physiologic occlusoapical movement of teeth. Therefore this treatment option should be used judiciously, mainly for mobile teeth that are already in jeopardy. Splinting of periodontally sound teeth should be done with extreme caution, if at all.

E. Esthetic repair of damaged or discolored teeth is routinely done with PFM restorations and represents one of the major developments in dentistry during the last 30 years. However, tooth preparation for PFM is the least conservative of all designs and significant pulpal and periodontal consequences usually follow improper technique. The guidelines for tooth preparation are well established. The PFM is viewed by many clinicians as the universal restoration; however, risk versus benefit analysis suggests that the dentist should recommend the most conservative technique that achieves the desired result. In some cases bleaching, veneering, or restoration of defects with composite resin may be the treatment of choice.

References

Shillingburg HT, Hobo S, Whitsett LD. Fundamentals of fixed prosthodontics. 2nd ed. Chicago: Quintessence Publishing, 1981:16.

Smith BGN. Dental crowns and bridges: Design and preparation. 2nd ed. Chicago: Year Book Medical Publishers, 1990:3, 135.

Stockstill JW, Bowley JF, Attanasio R. Clinical decision analysis in fixed prosthodontics. Dent Clin North Am 1992; 36:569.

Patient with UNSERVICEABLE RESTORATIONS, MISSING TEETH, OR ESTHETIC COMPROMISE

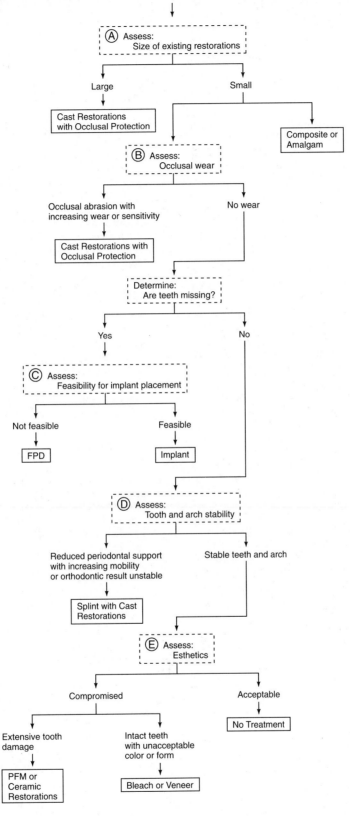

TREATMENT DECISIONS FOR FIXED PARTIAL DENTURES

Hugo Schmidt III

Although there is increasing recognition of implant therapy in the treatment of partial edentulism, the conventional fixed partial denture (FPD) remains the standard due to its established clinical success record and universal application. The fixed partial denture is not a conservative technique, and planning decisions, as well as prerestorative treatment, can profoundly affect the prognosis for an FPD. The indications for the various tooth replacement therapies overlap, and a careful, logical assessment of the patient's condition and desires is always needed.

A. The initial assessment is of the edentulous span and the functional requirements in the area. Ante's Law states that the root surface area of the supporting teeth should equal or exceed that of the teeth to be replaced, placing practical limits on span length in a fixed prosthesis. This law is violated regularly and successfully, depending on the location of the restoration. Three to four consecutively missing teeth are the maximum that can be replaced by a conventional FPD. Longer spans or distal extension edentulous areas should be restored by a removable partial denture (RPD) or implants. Carefully evaluate the functional burden in the area of treatment. Documented parafunctional habits, disrupted occlusal schemes, or replacement of guidance teeth increase the load on an FPD as well as demand for mechanical strength and abutment support.

B. The teeth adjacent to the edentulous space must be evaluated for their potential as abutment teeth. A number of factors related to length and firmness of the root, length of crown, axial alignment, and dental status must be reviewed before a prognosis can be determined for the prospective restoration. In situations where the abutment teeth have adequate supportive qualities but are improperly aligned or are coronally too short, adjunctive therapy such as orthodontics and surgical crown lengthening can make an unfavorable situation acceptable. When abutment teeth lack adequate bone support or are mobile, the approach must be to reinforce the abutment by including others through splinting. In a borderline situation a risk versus benefit analysis helps the dentist determine whether to proceed with a fixed prosthesis or to pursue alternative treatment modes.

C. The esthetic possibilities of restoring an anterior edentulous space must be evaluated before deciding upon an FPD. In the case of severely resorbed ridge or a high lip line, the social display of long pontic teeth may be unacceptable to the patient. If the ridge can be augmented to reduce pontic length to normal proportions, an FPD may still be indicated. Otherwise, another approach incorporating soft tissue in an RPD or implant restoration should be selected.

References

Johnson GK, Leary JM. Pontic design and localized ridge augmentation in fixed partial denture design. Dent Clin North Am 1992; 36:591.

Shillingburg HT, Hobo S, Whitsett LD. Fundamentals of fixed prosthodontics. 2nd ed. Chicago: Quintessence Publishing, 1981:13.

Smith DE. Interim dentures and treatment dentures. Dent Clin North Am 1984; 28:135.

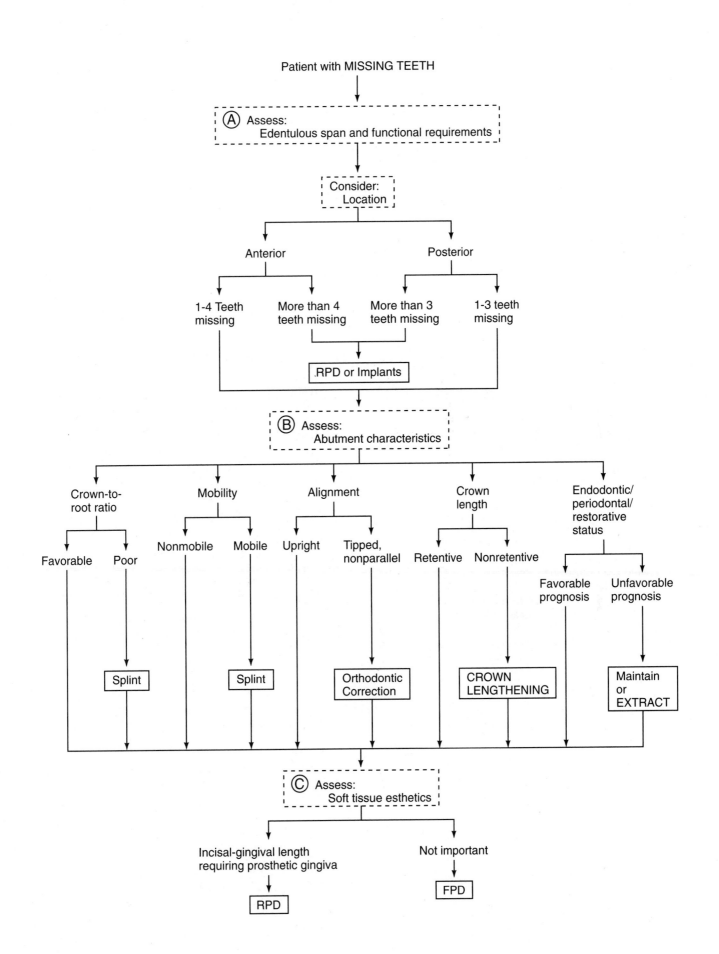

OCCLUSION

Eugene E. LaBarre

Excessive occlusal stress may be harmful to individual teeth or to the entire stomatognathic system. Reconstruction of major portions of a patient's occlusion is a time-consuming and demanding procedure. The problems caused by occlusal disharmony, as well as the advantages of an optimal occlusion, have been studied extensively. The well-established principles of simultaneous nondeflective centric contacts and smooth anterior group or canine guidance in eccentric movements should be incorporated in every occlusal reconstruction.

A. If the patient presents with signs and symptoms of temporomandibular dysfunction (TMD), comprehensive evaluation is necessary. Dental problems, such as occlusal stress, may be only a cofactor in TMD. Treatment protocols place the most conservative therapies first; occlusal reconstruction, if necessary, should be delayed until the symptoms of TMD have been eliminated or reduced to tolerable levels by reversible procedures. (The restorative dentist treating these patients is advised to work with health professionals knowledgeable about TMD or with a multidisciplinary TMD clinic.)

B. Most patients should have missing teeth replaced, not only to restore occlusal function but also to eliminate the potential for tooth migration and consequent occlusal instability. Conventional or implant-supported FPD and RPD are tooth replacement restorations.

C. Mild occlusal disharmony caused by premature centric contact or inappropriate guidance of mandibular movement may be corrected by selective grinding. More substantial problems require occlusal coverage restorations or orthodontic correction. Use articulated diagnostic casts to help determine the severity of the disharmony. In cases requiring multidisciplinary treatment, no rule applies concerning who performs the equilibration, but there should be agreement on the sequence and desired result.

D. Worn functional surfaces of teeth may be due to abrasion, attrition, or erosion. The cause of the problem should be identified. Conservative and reversible therapy, such as the occlusal splint and biofeedback, can reduce the rate of tooth wear but cannot permanently replace missing structures. Conservative therapy is indicated for mild wear cases or for maintaining restored occlusions. More severe tooth wear, involving thermal or contact sensitivity or esthetic compromise, must be restored with cemented restorations. The most extreme situations require a decision between heroic treatment, including endodontic treatment and surgical crown lengthening, or extraction followed by prosthetic treatment. In patients with extreme occlusal wear, the loss of vertical dimension may not be a certainty. These patients should be carefully evaluated, because increase of vertical dimension of occlusion beyond physiologic limits can cause severe and chronic problems.

References

Carranza FA. Glickman's clinical periodontology. 7th ed. Philadelphia: WB Saunders, 1990:73.

Dawson PE. Evaluation, diagnosis, and treatment of occlusal problems. St Louis: Mosby–Year Book, 1989:14.

Ramfjord S, Ash MM. Occlusion. 3rd ed. Philadelphia: WB Saunders, 1983:459.

Shillingburg HT, Hobo S, Whitsett LD. Fundamentals of fixed prosthodontics. 2nd ed. Chicago: Quintessence Publishing, 1981:17.

Patient for OCCLUSAL EVALUATION

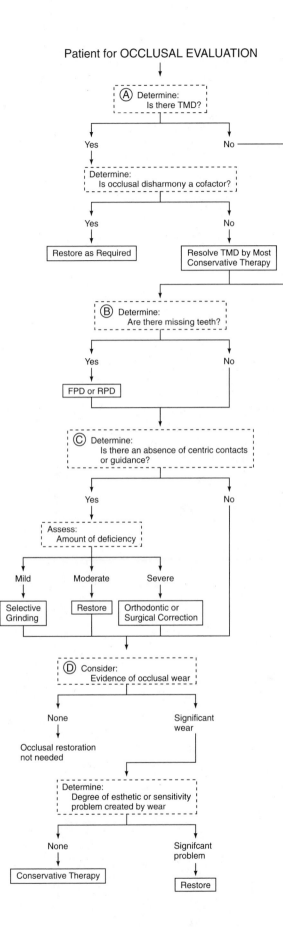

PROVISIONAL REMOVABLE PARTIAL DENTURE

Eugene E. LaBarre

The provisional removable partial denture (RPD) is an interim all-acrylic prosthesis with wire clasps. It is useful to provide esthetic or functional restoration of missing teeth during the time required for postextraction healing or for complex treatment. It can be used to evaluate occlusion, esthetics, or other treatment outcomes when the prognosis is uncertain. The main advantages of the "treatment" RPD are ease and low cost of fabrication, application to most restorative situations, and ability to modify the prosthesis as needed during multidisciplinary treatment.

A. Often, in complex restorative cases, the long-term goals of treatment may be hidden or complicated by the patient's acute needs. If removable restorations already exist, they may be unacceptable or difficult to maintain during treatment. A provisional RPD would also benefit a patient who requires extraction of teeth in the esthetic zone or whose occlusal function will be severely handicapped by posterior extractions. In these situations the provisional RPD is inserted immediately at the time of the extractions.

B. Fabrication of a "treatment" RPD is a simple laboratory process that requires only mounted diagnostic casts and a tooth shade from the dentist. In situations of tight interdigitation between opposing teeth, a proximal groove may be necessary to permit space for a wire clasp. If long-term use of the provisional RPD is expected, rests can be incorporated on abutment teeth.

C. If the provisional RPD has been inserted immediately after extractions, denture liners may be used periodically to maintain intimacy of fit with the healing soft tissues. Other phases of treatment can begin when the patient has adapted to the new restoration. If the definitive restoration involves an RPD of similar outline, the provisional prosthesis can be permanently relined as a spare.

References

Weintraub GS. Provisional removable partial and complete prostheses. Dent Clin North Amer 1989; 33:399.

Yalisove IL. Selected cases to illustrate versatility of provisional removable prostheses. Dent Clin North Am 1989; 33:531.

Patient with MULTIPLE, EXTENSIVE DENTAL PROBLEMS

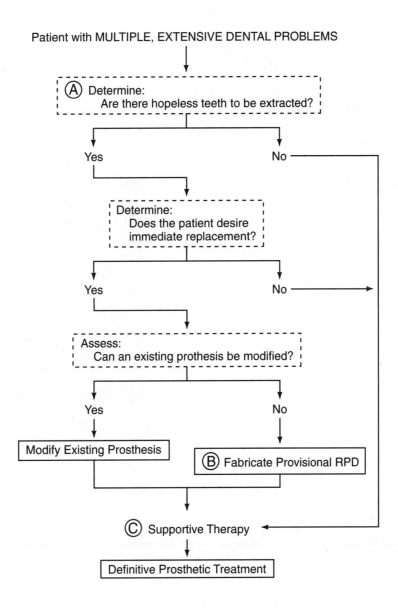

RAPID EXTRUSION VERSUS CROWN LENGTHENING SURGERY

Kathy I. Mueller
Galen W. Wagnild

Salvage of teeth severely compromised by caries, fracture, or large defective restorations often depends on the extent of damage below the free gingival margin. A tooth lengthening procedure is required when significant structural degradation has occurred. Periodontal crown lengthening surgery is a one step tooth lengthening procedure that can expose most defects for restorative correction. This approach removes soft and hard supporting tissues and moves the attachment level apically. The tooth position remains unchanged; however, this surgery may affect esthetics and/or the maintenance potential of adjacent teeth. Rapid orthodontic extrusion is an alternative tooth lengthening method that also facilitates restoration of compromised teeth. This procedure moves the residual tooth structure coronally while the soft and hard supporting tissues remain in their pretreatment locations. Orthodontic rapid extrusion is indicated when esthetic considerations are critical or when adjacent tooth anatomy and adjacent coronal restorations would be jeopardized by the surgical apical repositioning of periodontal tissues.

A. To be successful over time, restorative procedures must not invade the attachment apparatus. There must be adequate sound tooth structure between the lesion and the coronal extent of the junctional epithelium to place a restorative margin. The margin generally requires 2 mm of sound tooth structure coronal to the attachment. Operative invasion of the attachment often results in gingival recession, periodontal pocket formation, or chronic gingival inflammation (Fig. 1).

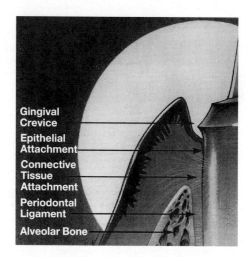

Figure 1. The restorative margin must terminate on sound tooth structure coronal to the epithelial attachment. Mutilated teeth require alteration of the tooth/attachment relationship prior to restoration. This modification will allow margin placement while maintaining the integrity of the attachment apparatus.

Gingival Crevice
Epithelial Attachment
Connective Tissue Attachment
Periodontal Ligament
Alveolar Bone

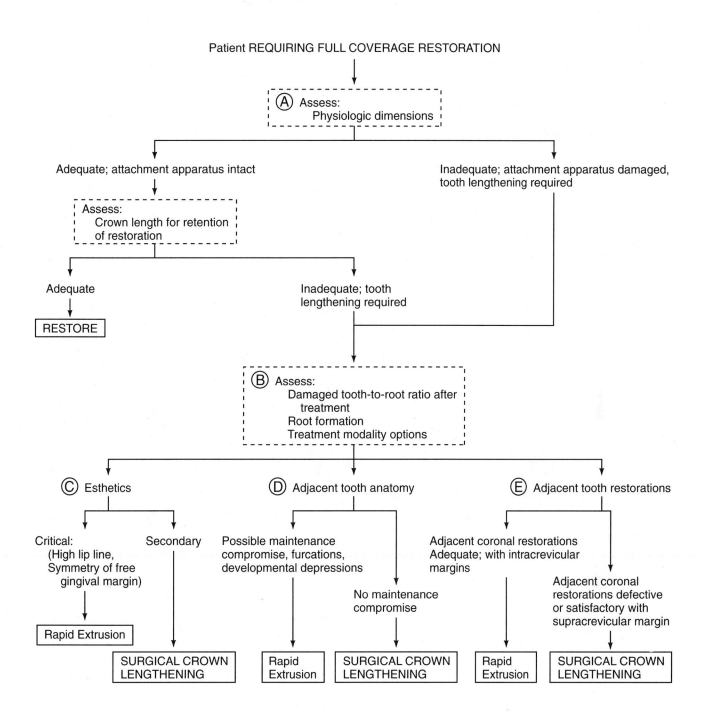

Patient REQUIRING FULL COVERAGE RESTORATION

Ⓐ Assess:
Physiologic dimensions

Adequate; attachment apparatus intact

Inadequate; attachment apparatus damaged, tooth lengthening required

Assess:
Crown length for retention
of restoration

Adequate

RESTORE

Inadequate; tooth
lengthening required

Ⓑ Assess:
Damaged tooth-to-root ratio after
treatment
Root formation
Treatment modality options

Ⓒ Esthetics

Ⓓ Adjacent tooth anatomy

Ⓔ Adjacent tooth restorations

Critical:
(High lip line,
Symmetry of free
gingival margin)

Secondary

Possible maintenance
compromise, furcations,
developmental depressions

Adjacent coronal restorations
Adequate; with intracrevicular
margins

Rapid Extrusion

SURGICAL CROWN
LENGTHENING

No maintenance
compromise

Adjacent coronal
restorations defective
or satisfactory with
supracrevicular margin

Rapid
Extrusion

SURGICAL CROWN
LENGTHENING

Rapid
Extrusion

SURGICAL CROWN
LENGTHENING

B. Retention of the severely damaged tooth requires critical pretreatment evaluation. Accurate prediction of posttreatment crown-to-root ratio is mandatory. Sufficient periodontal attachment for the tooth to withstand functional forces must remain after the procedure. With all other variables equal rapid orthodontic extrusion provides a more favorable posttreatment crown-to-root ratio than does periodontal crown lengthening surgery.

Cylindrical root form greatly enhances the functional and esthetic components of tooth lengthening. A tapered root form compromises the remaining periodontal ligament attachment after either procedure. Likewise, gingival embrasures are exaggerated when either orthodontics or surgery is performed on a tapered root (Fig. 2).

C. Esthetic variables have a great impact on the modality selection between rapid orthodontic extrusion and periodontal crown lengthening surgery. Patients with great esthetic expectations and a high lip line may not tolerate the deformity produced by surgery. This defect will be apparent on the damaged tooth as well as adjacent teeth, in most cases.

Maintenance of free gingival margin symmetry could dictate that surgery be expanded to include the entire anterior sextant. This surgical expansion exposes root structure on all included teeth. These significant sequelae may be avoided by using orthodontics to correct the defect (Fig. 2).

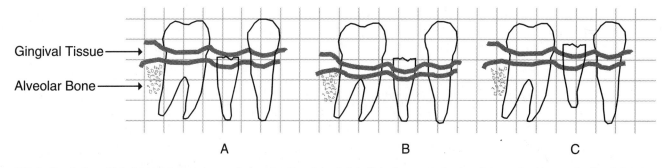

Gingival Tissue

Alveolar Bone

A   B   C

Figure 2. **A**, A mutilated second premolar requires restoration; there is insufficient coronal structure for margin placement without damage to the attachment mechanism. **B**, Surgical crown lengthening exposes sufficient sound tooth structure; the periodontal tissues are apically repositioned and the root position is unchanged. **C**, Orthodontic extrusion exposes sufficient sound tooth structure; the periodontal tissue position is unchanged but the root has been repositioned coronally.

D. The selected modality should not solve one problem while creating others. Short root trunks or significant developmental grooves on adjacent teeth may be exposed by surgery and therefore require the damaged tooth to be extruded. These anatomic findings render a tooth more difficult to maintain if the attachment level is moved apically by a surgical technique (Fig. 2).

E. Existing coronal restorations on adjacent teeth also influence the selection of extrusion or surgery. Intracrevicular margins on adjacent teeth are exposed by conventional periodontal surgical techniques to lengthen the tooth. Restorations that do not need replacement and demand intracrevicular margins for esthetics are indications for orthodontic rapid extrusion of the damaged tooth (Fig. 2).

References

Biggerstaff R, Sinks J, Carazola J. Orthodontic extrusion and biologic width realignment procedures: Methods for reclaiming nonrestorable teeth. J Am Dent Assoc 1986; 112:345.

Kozlovsky A, Tal H, Lieberman M. Forced eruption combined with gingival fiberectomy. A technique for crown lengthening. J Clin Periodontol 1988; 15:534.

Pontoriero R, Celenza F, Ricci G, Carnevale G. Rapid extrusion with fiber resection: A combined orthodontic-periodontal treatment modality. Int J Periodont Restor Dent 1987; 5:30.

Rosenberg E, Garber D, Evian C. Tooth lengthening procedures. Compend Contin Educ 1980; 1(3):161.

SUPRAGINGIVAL VERSUS INTRACREVICULAR MARGIN PLACEMENT

Kathy I. Mueller
Galen W. Wagnild

The marginal periodontium operated on daily by restorative dentists requires definitive, logical decisions regarding margin location. Literature supports placement of margins slightly into the crevice or coronal to the free gingival margin. Restorations located deep in the sulcus risk irreversible damage to the supporting structures.

A. Esthetic requirements may dictate intracrevicular margin location despite other clinical findings that would allow a supragingival location. It is important to determine esthetic margin placement using factors such as tooth position, visibility of the margin area during normal function and the patient's understanding of the objectives of the restorative therapy. The margin of a porcelain fused to metal restoration often can be placed 0.5 to 1.0 mm into a healthy gingival crevice. In a thin, scalloped gingival architecture, it may be impossible to conceal a metal collar margin at this depth. This problem may be resolved by use of a porcelain shoulder margin or a margin supported by metal that does not display a visible collar. When esthetics are secondary and structural features permit, restorative margins can be located outside of the gingival crevice. Supragingival margins are more accurately prepared, more predictably recorded, and more accessible for evaluation, finishing, and patient maintenance.

B. Adequate preparation length to retain the final restoration must be planned. In cases with marginally adequate coronal structure, an additional 1 mm of axial wall can often be obtained by preparing within the gingival crevice. The physiologic zone or biologic width must be maintained intact (Fig. 1). Attempts to increase coverage by apically positioning the restorative margin are limited by this fragile complex. Violation of this width may result in chronic gingival inflammation, recession of the free gingival margin, loss of crestal bone and pocket formation. If adequate retention and resistance cannot be obtained within the parameters of a healthy periodontium, surgical crown lengthening or rapid orthodontic extrusion may be indicated. Patients requiring restoration after periodontal therapy pose additional complexities. The gingival attachment is often positioned more apically and postsurgical cases may have very shallow gingival sulci. Attempts to place margins within the sulcus may lead to breakdown of the tissue complex. The elongated clinical crown in the periodontally compromised case requires additional axial wall reduction to achieve intracrevicular margins. This preparation may encroach on the pulp and threaten the vitality of the tooth. When possible, postsurgical margins should be placed above the free gingival margin.

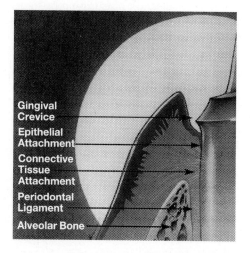

Figure 1. The restorative margin must terminate above the level of the epithelial attachment. Potential operative damage and greater maintenance difficulty can occur as the margin approaches the base of the gingival crevice.

C. Preparation of margins should extend beyond existing restorations and lesions onto sound tooth structure. This sound structure should be a minimum of 2 mm in height. Placement of the margin in the gingival crevice will often accomplish these goals. However, defects deep in the crevice or into the attachment apparatus should be treated with surgical crown lengthening or orthodontic extrusion.

D. Root sensitivity may be controlled or eliminated by conservative means. In severe cases endodontic treatment may be required. Supragingival margin placement is suggested if root sensitivity has been resolved prior to restoration.

References

Nevins M, Skurow H. The intracrevicular restorative margin, the biologic width, and maintenance of the gingival margin. Int J Periodont Restor Dent 1984; 3:31.

Schluger S, Yuodelis R, Page R, Johnson R. Periodontal diseases: Basic phenomena, clinical management and occlusal and restorative interrelationships. Philadelphia: Lea & Febiger, 1990.

Shillingburg H, Hobo S, Whitsett D. Fundamentals of fixed prosthodontics. 2nd ed. Berlin: Quintessence Publishing, 1981:79.

Wilson R, Maynard G. Intracrevicular restorative dentistry. Int J Periodont Restor Dent 1981; 4:35.

Patient with a TOOTH REQUIRING A FULL COVERAGE RESTORATION

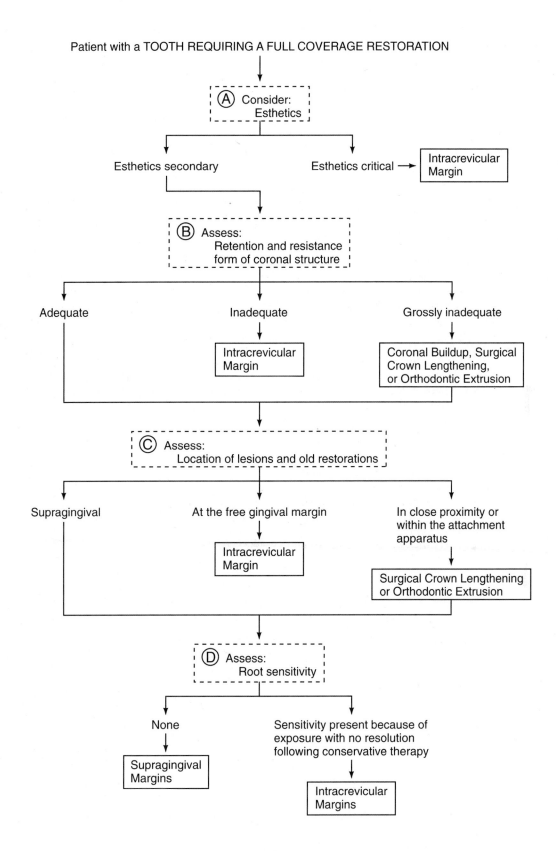

(A) Consider:
Esthetics

Esthetics secondary   Esthetics critical → Intracrevicular Margin

(B) Assess:
Retention and resistance
form of coronal structure

Adequate   Inadequate   Grossly inadequate

Intracrevicular Margin   Coronal Buildup, Surgical Crown Lengthening, or Orthodontic Extrusion

(C) Assess:
Location of lesions and old restorations

Supragingival   At the free gingival margin   In close proximity or within the attachment apparatus

Intracrevicular Margin   Surgical Crown Lengthening or Orthodontic Extrusion

(D) Assess:
Root sensitivity

None   Sensitivity present because of exposure with no resolution following conservative therapy

Supragingival Margins   Intracrevicular Margins

DETERMINING THE NEED TO SPLINT

Chi Tran

Several restorative situations may require groups of teeth to be reinforced by splinting them together, either by temporary or permanent means.

A. The initial evaluation should determine the periodontal status of the involved teeth. Soft tissue inflammation in an environment of reduced alveolar support and heavy functional demands leads to more bone loss, increasing mobility and loss of teeth. If periodontal treatment is likely to fail, permanent forms of splinting should not be attempted because little advantage can be attained for the patient. Arrested or successfully treated periodontitis lends itself to a variety of restorative options.

B. Tooth mobility patterns must be evaluated in the context of past records and future expectations. Teeth with documented increasing mobility patterns are unstable and may be expected to continually worsen until they are no longer serviceable. In the absence of inflammatory disease a good prognosis can be achieved in these cases by mechanically splinting the loose tooth to strong neighbors or by splinting weak adjacent teeth to each other. A variety of splinting operations are possible (e.g., removable appliances, intermediate techniques utilizing composite resin and wire splints, and definitive procedures such as soldered cast gold or porcelain fused to metal restorations). Splinting techniques embody a wide range of technical difficulty and expense. They should be selected following a deliberate risk versus benefit analysis.

C. Uncontrolled drifting and migration of teeth may be caused by a number of factors: periodontal disease, tooth loss, unstable orthodontic results, or occlusal trauma. Instability of anterior teeth is often reported by patients; posterior tooth movement must be deduced from patterns of extrusion, drifting, and collapse. In most situations splinting can only intercept tooth movement patterns; definitive realignment must be accomplished orthodontically or surgically.

D. Occasionally, teeth must be reinforced because of exceptional occlusal demands or because they must support fixed or removable prostheses. In these situations the restorative dentist must accurately predict the number of reinforcement teeth that are required to withstand the load. Double abutting and cross-arch splinting are acceptable techniques for increasing the support of long span restorations.

References

Dawson PE. Evaluation, diagnosis, and treatment of occlusal problems. St Louis: Mosby—Year Book, 1989:483.

Ramfjord S, Ash MM. Occlusion. 3rd ed. Philadelphia: WB Saunders, 1983:481.

Smith BGN. Dental crowns and bridges: Design and preparation. 2nd ed. Chicago: Year Book Medical Publishers, 1990:211.

Patient with TEETH WITH REDUCED BONE SUPPORT

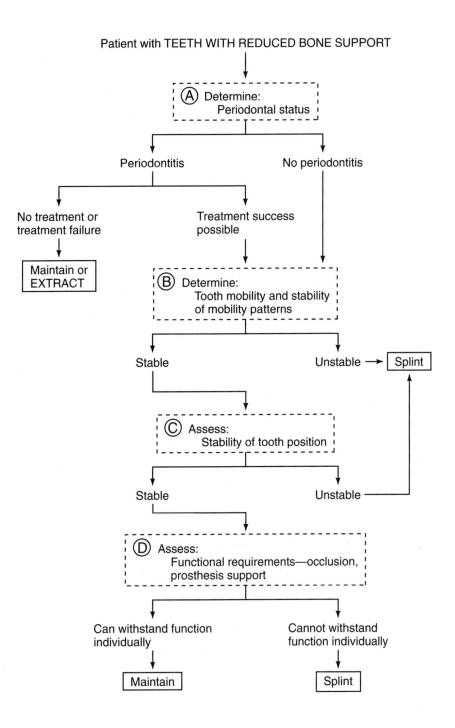

TELESCOPIC PROSTHESES VERSUS CONVENTIONAL APPROACHES

Eugene E. LaBarre

Telescopic prostheses are two component restorations. The prepared teeth are covered with cast metal copings that provide marginal seal and ideally tapered axial surfaces. A fixed partial denture (FPD) or removable overdenture is supported by the copings.

A. In a patient with misaligned abutment teeth, copings can be placed to realign axial surfaces to a common path of insertion. Examples of conditions that may defy orthodontic correction include atypical dental development associated with severe cleft palate or partial anodontia associated with dentinogenesis imperfecta. An FPD or removable overdenture may be placed on the parallel copings.

B. The most common application of telescopic restorations is in periodontal prostheses. In these cases, periodontal support is compromised and teeth with uncertain long-term prognosis may be required as splinted abutments. The telescopic FPD is considered a reversible restoration, because it is luted with provisional cement. This permits removal for periodic maintenance or when an abutment must be extracted. This technically demanding procedure requires sub-stantial tooth reduction to avoid overcontouring associated with double margins and two restorations on each abutment tooth.

C. If the patient profile permits and there is bone of sufficient quantity and quality to support implants, heroic salvage of periodontally compromised teeth may be less predictable and less satisfactory to the patient than implant treatment. However, telescopic restorations are preferred to complete dentures for those patients who will not consider implants. The patient should understand the heroic nature of telescopic restorations, should demonstrate adequate home care, and participate in periodic recall. Patient cooperation is the most critical determinant of success in these complex treatment modalities.

References

Shillingburg HT, Hobo S, Whitsett LD. Fundamentals of fixed prosthodontics. 2nd ed. Chicago: Quintessence Publishing, 1981:32.

Yalisove IL, Dietz JB. Telescopic prosthetic therapy. Philadelphia: GF Stickley, 1977:7.

Patient for EXTENSIVE RESTORATIVE TREATMENT

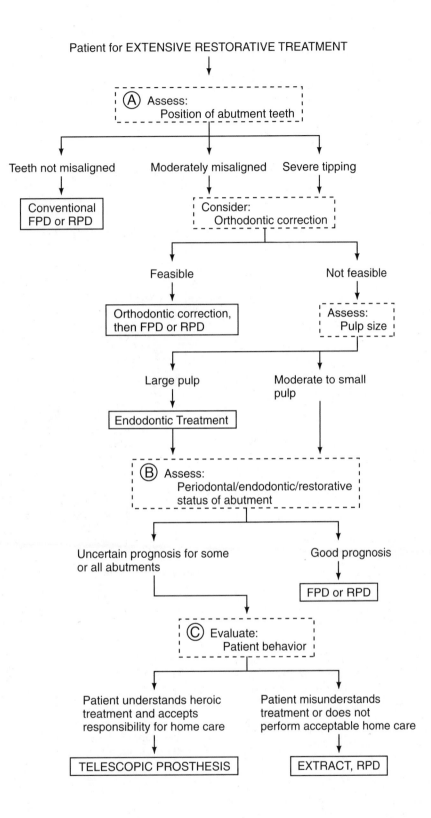

Ⓐ Assess:
   Position of abutment teeth

Teeth not misaligned   Moderately misaligned   Severe tipping

Conventional
FPD or RPD

Consider:
   Orthodontic correction

Feasible   Not feasible

Orthodontic correction,
then FPD or RPD

Assess:
   Pulp size

Large pulp   Moderate to small
pulp

Endodontic Treatment

Ⓑ Assess:
   Periodontal/endodontic/restorative
   status of abutment

Uncertain prognosis for some
or all abutments   Good prognosis

FPD or RPD

Ⓒ Evaluate:
   Patient behavior

Patient understands heroic
treatment and accepts
responsibility for home care

Patient misunderstands
treatment or does not
perform acceptable home care

TELESCOPIC PROSTHESIS   EXTRACT, RPD

ADHESIVE FIXED PARTIAL DENTURE VERSUS CONVENTIONAL PROSTHETICS

Eugene E. LaBarre

Adhesive fixed partial dentures (A-FPDs) differ from conventional FPDs in that tooth preparation and retainer design are more conservative, mechanical or chemical adhesive mechanisms are required for both tooth structure and the internal aspect of the retainers, and an adhesive resin is used as a luting medium. Clinical research has demonstrated that A-FPDs are associated with an extremely low incidence of recurrent caries, periodontal inflammation, and patient dissatisfaction. The main problem with an A-FPD is partial or complete debonding of the restoration from the abutment teeth; the incidence varies from study to study but is significantly greater than that for conventional FPD (Fig. 1).

A. The A-FPD is a simple restoration and should be used to replace single missing teeth only (two mandibular incisors may be acceptable). Replacing multiple missing teeth or use of multiple abutments should be avoided. The abutment teeth should be intact and sturdy. The strength of the bond is determined by surface area of retainer coverage; mobility in abutments significantly increases fatigue of the bond. For this reason, adhesive splints involving multiple mobile teeth are discouraged because they have shown high incidence of debonding and it is difficult or impossible to repair a partially debonded splint.

B. Patients with parafunctional habits have lower success rates with A-FPD. Constant and forceful clenching or bruxing cause fatigue failure of the bond. For similar reasons, restoration of lateral guidance (e.g., replacement of a maxillary canine) should be avoided. The ideal patient for the A-FPD has uniform nondeflective centric contacts and effective anterior guidance.

C. For anterior restorations, centric and guiding contacts should be located in the incisal third, permitting the gingival two-thirds to be covered by the retainer without interfering with occlusion. Deep anterior occlusion is the most common contraindication for anterior A-FPD. The situation that most favors longevity of an A-FPD is the anterior open bite; however, in these cases the dental technician must be advised not to cover the incisal edge with metal to avoid creating a gray color in the abutment teeth. This phenomenon is notoriously difficult to predict and is best avoided by leaving the incisal edge uncovered. For the same reason, caution must be exercised when using thin incisors as abutments, because they may appear much darker after luting the restoration. Once graying has occurred, the only solution is to remove the restoration, which involves tedious ultrasonic vibration or sectioning of each retainer.

Diminished width of tooth space is a common finding in adults who lost an anterior tooth during

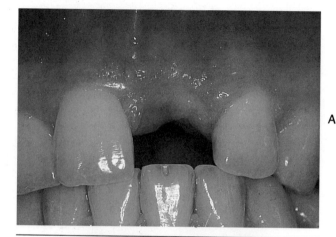

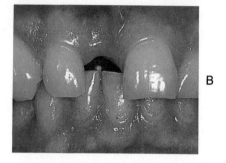

Figure 1. Preoperative presentation of candidates for A-FPD. **A,** Good indications for A-FPD: centric occlusion in incisal one third, unblemished abutment teeth, edentulous ridge, and space within normal limits. **B,** Poor indications for A-FPD: excessive vertical overlap and edentulous space that is narrow mesiodistally.

childhood. Many of these individuals have used an acrylic stayplate or flipper for many years. The appearance of these "temporary" restorations is a good indication of whether a PFM pontic can satisfy the individual's esthetic demands. In cases of slightly diminished width the abutment teeth can be narrowed during tooth preparation. Solutions for moderately reduced space include lapping the pontic facially over one or both abutments or conventional FPD. Severely reduced spaces may require orthodontic correction.

D. Finally, the patient should be informed about the potential for debonding to occur within the first 5 years of service and should be willing to accept the consequences of a partial debonded restoration. The patient should also be informed about alternative approaches.

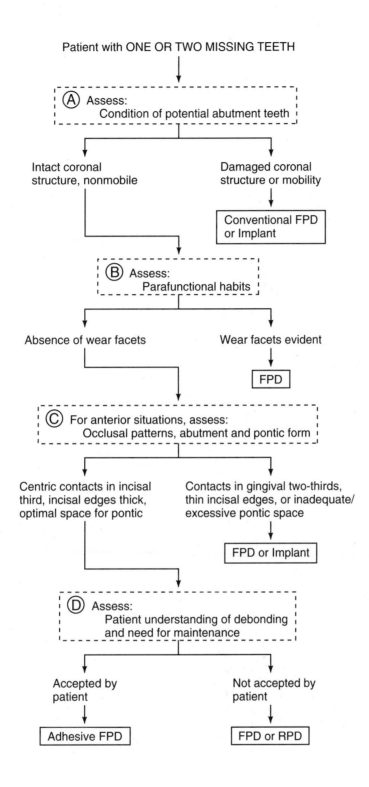

Patient with ONE OR TWO MISSING TEETH

Ⓐ Assess:
Condition of potential abutment teeth

Intact coronal
structure, nonmobile

Damaged coronal
structure or mobility

Conventional FPD
or Implant

Ⓑ Assess:
Parafunctional habits

Absence of wear facets

Wear facets evident

FPD

Ⓒ For anterior situations, assess:
Occlusal patterns, abutment and pontic form

Centric contacts in incisal
third, incisal edges thick,
optimal space for pontic

Contacts in gingival two-thirds,
thin incisal edges, or inadequate/
excessive pontic space

FPD or Implant

Ⓓ Assess:
Patient understanding of debonding
and need for maintenance

Accepted by
patient

Not accepted by
patient

Adhesive FPD

FPD or RPD

References

Creugers NH, et al. An analysis of clinical studies on resin-bonded bridges. J Dent Res 1991; 70:146.

Simonsen R, Thompson V, Barrack G. Etch cast restorations: Clinical and laboratory techniques. Chicago: Quintessence Publishing, 1983.

ENDODONTIC EFFECTS OF CAST RESTORATIONS

Eugene E. LaBarre

Pulpal sensitivity is a common complaint following fixed prosthodontic procedures on vital teeth. Except for obvious situations, such as preparing virgin teeth with large pulps or overpreparing because of occlusal or path of insertion demands, development of pulpal symptoms is difficult to predict and may seem to occur in random patterns in prosthodontic practice. The clinician should be familiar with possible etiologies of pulpal trauma and exercise universal precautions to reduce its occurrence.

A. During tooth preparation for full coverage restorations, potential for significant damage to the pulp exists. The enamel is removed, and all of the dentinal tubules in the coronal aspect of the tooth are cut. Overheating is the most common source of postoperative sensitivity, and the clinician should always monitor the amount of water spray and cutting efficiency of diamonds and burs. Clogged or worn rotary instruments should be replaced. Other contributing factors include: excessive pressure during grinding, vibration from asymmetric rotary instruments, and desiccation to aid visibility and impression making. Routine use of a dentin bonding agent or unfilled resin is recommended immediately following completion of tooth preparation to seal dentinal tubules and to protect the pulp from further trauma.

The provisional restoration must be managed with care, also. If large amounts of acrylic resin are polymerized directly on the prepared teeth, the exothermic setting reaction can cause a substantial increase in intrapulpal temperature. Frequent pumping and cooling of the provisional restoration are necessary during polymerization. Attention to fit is also important to minimize the effects of microleakage and occlusal trauma.

The cementation process has been shown to irritate a vital pulp. A barrier in the form of copal varnish or bonding agent is recommended. Cements differ in their capacities to elicit pulpal response. This has proven difficult to evaluate through clinical trials. As with tooth preparation, the clinician should realize that the luting procedure is a critical step for the health of the vital pulp and universal precautions should be exercised to minimize trauma to the pulp.

Thermal shock continues to be a significant problem following cementation of cast restorations. General recommendations include placing a base on deep areas of tooth preparation and advising patients that the situation is usually transient.

A tooth restored by a cast restoration may develop symptoms after long periods of comfort. Such cases usually suggest a chronic inflammatory response in the pulp that is clinically unremarkable until an exacerbation initiates symptoms. The pulpal status may result from the cumulative insult of previous caries and several restorative procedures. If obvious factors (e.g., occlusal trauma, recurrent decay, or fractures) are not found, no treatment is indicated until symptoms warrant endodontic therapy.

B. Mild pulpal symptoms (e.g., thermal sensitivity that disappears when the stimulant is removed) indicate reversible pulpitis. No treatment is indicated in these situations until symptoms worsen.

C. Severe symptoms (e.g., unprovoked pain, throbbing that interrupts sleep, or pain that lingers after the stimulus is removed) are more ominous and suggest irreversible pulpitis. Endodontic therapy is indicated.

D. Restored teeth with severe pulpal symptoms should be evaluated for vertical periodontal defects to rule out a cracked root. If a crack is detected, heroic treatment involving endodontic therapy and periodontal maintenance of the defect area is unpredictable. In many cases extraction is the only effective treatment for the pain associated with these teeth.

References

Cohen S, Burns RC. Pathways of the pulp. 5th ed. St Louis: Mosby—Year Book, 1991:434.

Shillingburg HT, Hobo S, Whitsett LD. Fundamentals of fixed prosthodontics. 2nd ed. Chicago: Quintessence Publishing, 1981:161, 379.

Patient with PULPAL SYMPTOMS FOLLOWING RESTORATION OF A VITAL TOOTH

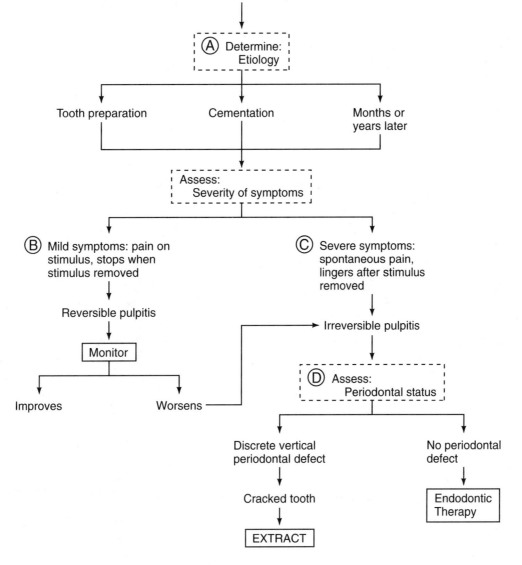

ORAL CONDITIONS THAT MAY REQUIRE PREPROSTHETIC SURGERY

Eugene E. LaBarre

A patient who presents for prosthetic treatment must be examined carefully to assure that the residual ridges are or will be in an optimal condition to support dentures. A variety of hard and soft tissue conditions interfere with intimate fit between oral tissue and prosthesis and may require surgical repair. Any existing dentures should be examined to indicate whether and how the new prostheses might fit around the problem.

A. In cases that require extraction, soft tissue recontouring, and minor osseous reduction, the denture may be placed as an immediate restoration, using a temporary soft reliner to establish intimate fit and a seal, if necessary. Occasionally, extraction is followed by reduction of facially prominent bone or smoothing of interproximal bone spicules, although this should be minimized in favor of preserving the residual ridge.

B. Residual ridge resorption (RRR) is a particular problem for edentulous patients. In the past surgical treatment of RRR has included deepening the soft tissue vestibule or grafting ceramic or osseous materials to augment the ridge. These procedures are still performed, but they are as invasive as implant placement and do not insure significantly improved denture service. For this reason, augmentation procedures are more important to create adequate bone support for implants, more than to increase the denture-bearing area. At present, surgical augmentation for RRR is rapidly developing. Scientific data on the long-term success rates of augmented implants are lacking.

References

Fonseca RJ. Reconstructive preprosthetic oral and maxillofacial surgery. Philadelphia: WB Saunders, 1986.

Hopkins R. Preprosthetic oral surgery. Philadelphia: Lea & Febiger, 1987.

Pedersen GW. Oral surgery. Philadelphia: WB Saunders, 1988:119.

Zarb GA. Boucher's prosthodontic treatment for edentulous patients. 10th ed. St Louis: Mosby–Year Book, 1990: 123.

Patient requiring a REMOVABLE PROSTHESIS

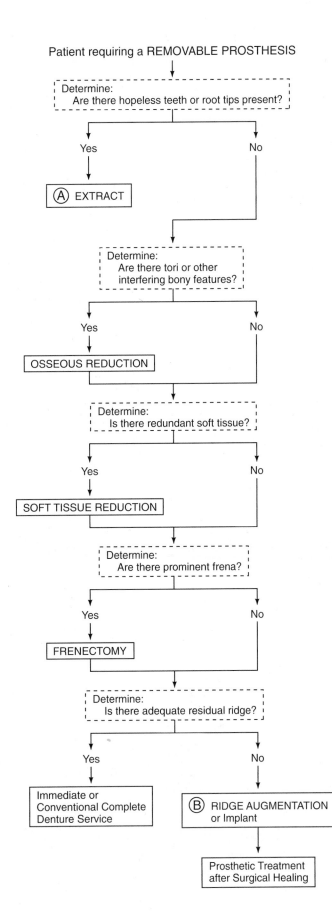

Determine:
Are there hopeless teeth or root tips present?

Yes → Ⓐ EXTRACT

No →

Determine:
Are there tori or other interfering bony features?

Yes → OSSEOUS REDUCTION

No →

Determine:
Is there redundant soft tissue?

Yes → SOFT TISSUE REDUCTION

No →

Determine:
Are there prominent frena?

Yes → FRENECTOMY

No →

Determine:
Is there adequate residual ridge?

Yes → Immediate or Conventional Complete Denture Service

No → Ⓑ RIDGE AUGMENTATION or Implant → Prosthetic Treatment after Surgical Healing

TRANSITION TO DENTURES FOR THE PATIENT WITH A HOPELESS DENTITION

Eugene E. LaBarre

Full mouth extraction and transition to complete dentures represent a treatment option for patients with severely compromised natural teeth. Most often, this option must be chosen because of extreme neglect and/or financial considerations. Also, for patients in whom periodontal or restorative therapy has failed, complete dentures may be the final treatment or may be used as a transition during implant therapy.

A. The first decision that should be made concerning a patient with hopeless dentition is whether the teeth should be removed immediately, before a transitional prosthesis is fabricated. Conditions that warrant this approach include severe dental infection or pain or teeth that are so mobile or malposed that impression making is impossible. In these situations the substantial health risk overrides esthetic or oral function considerations. Denture fabrication should be delayed 4 to 6 weeks postoperatively to permit healing and initial residual ridge remodeling. A conventional technique then can be used to restore function.

B. The number and condition of the teeth to be extracted determine the sequence of surgical procedures. The classical technique for immediate dentures involves removing the posterior teeth, waiting for suitable ridge remodeling, and then fabricating the dentures and delivering them when the anterior teeth are extracted. This technique requires that the anterior teeth be present and able to withstand several months of function between surgical phases. The advantage of the technique is that it permits placement of the denture on a mature posterior ridge, which reduces the need to reline at delivery and makes the initial service of the denture more predictable.

C. The most common way of managing the transitional denture is to fabricate the prosthesis first, often by a simplified technique, and to deliver it when all teeth are removed in a single surgery. Temporary resilient denture liners make this possible, because the fit of an immediate transitional denture can be customized very easily. Typically, the patient is maintained with temporary reliners until the ridge has been remodeled (3 to 6 months); the denture is then permanently relined.

D. If necessary, proceed with a second denture or begin implant treatment, during which the transitional denture continues to be used.

References

Weintraub GS. Provisional removable partial and complete prostheses. Dent Clin North Am 1989; 33:399.

Zarb GA. Boucher's prosthodontic treatment for edentulous patients. 10th ed. St Louis: Mosby—Year Book, 1990: 534.

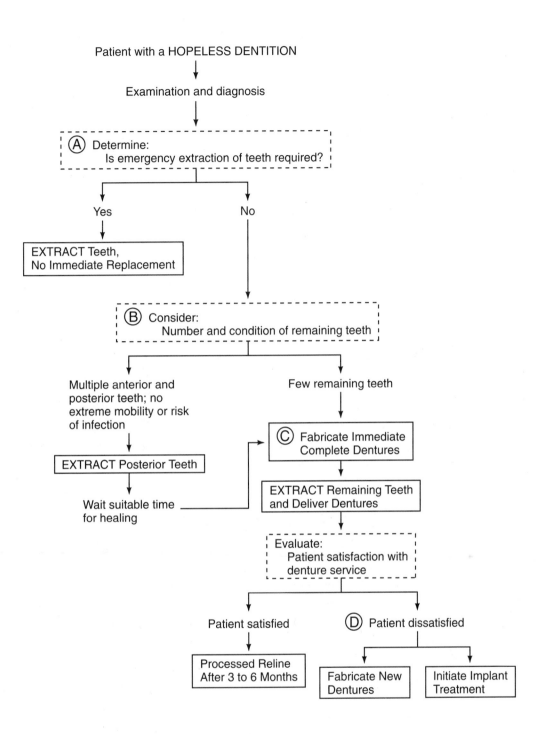

Patient with a HOPELESS DENTITION

Examination and diagnosis

(A) Determine:
Is emergency extraction of teeth required?

Yes — EXTRACT Teeth, No Immediate Replacement

No — (B) Consider: Number and condition of remaining teeth

Multiple anterior and posterior teeth; no extreme mobility or risk of infection — EXTRACT Posterior Teeth — Wait suitable time for healing

Few remaining teeth — (C) Fabricate Immediate Complete Dentures — EXTRACT Remaining Teeth and Deliver Dentures

Evaluate: Patient satisfaction with denture service

Patient satisfied — Processed Reline After 3 to 6 Months

(D) Patient dissatisfied — Fabricate New Dentures / Initiate Implant Treatment

REMOVABLE PARTIAL DENTURE DESIGN CONSIDERATIONS FOR THE PERIODONTALLY COMPROMISED PATIENT

Eugene E. LaBarre

Although the fixed partial denture (FPD) is the restoration of choice for restoring missing teeth, the removable partial denture (RPD) becomes necessary when the edentulous span is too long or when there is no end tooth (distal extension).

A. The need for tooth replacement is first assessed according to the patient's esthetic or functional disability. Not all partially edentulous patients require restoration; when all molars are missing, a well-integrated second premolar occlusion is satisfactory for many people.

B. When an RPD is fabricated for a periodontally compromised patient, the prosthesis should fit well, be rigid, and result in minimal coverage of marginal gingiva by the metallic portion. Open major connector designs placed at least 3 mm apical to marginal tissue in the mandible (6 mm in the maxilla) are preferred over plated designs, which cover the lingual surfaces of multiple teeth.

C. Edentulous areas that are capable of supporting occlusal loads are covered fully, particularly in distal extension situations. The altered cast impression technique provides soft tissue contact simultaneous with seating of the rests, minimizing rocking of the restoration in function. A variety of mechanical clasping systems have been described to reduce functional leverage-type forces on distal extension RPD abutments (Fig. 1). If precision attachments are desirable esthetically, resilient designs that permit tissue-ward movement and rotation are necessary for periodontally compromised abutments.

D. Splinting is required to reinforce mobile RPD abutments and is strongly recommended for free-standing premolar pier abutments. Double abutting also may be necessary for nonmobile abutments adjacent to severely resorbed distal extension residual ridges because of the potential for increased movement of the restoration and consequent damage to the abutment teeth. The presence of six or fewer anterior teeth as the only support in the arch for an RPD is a common occurrence. In this situation splinting all the teeth offers excellent support for the RPD. Highly mobile teeth have little value as RPD abutments and should be extracted. There must be at least two strategic nonmobile abutments or abutment groups to support an RPD; otherwise, a complete denture is indicated.

E. The optimal occlusion for the reduced support RPD involves uniform posterior centric contacts without significant laterally displacing forces. Natural tooth guidance, if it exists and is nondestructive, should be maintained. Prosthetic tooth materials should have wear properties compatible with those of opposing dentition to preserve occlusal contact patterns: acrylic opposite acrylic; metal opposite enamel, metal, or porcelain fused to metal; and porcelain opposite porcelain denture teeth.

The success of any restoration in a compromised oral scheme depends on effective home care and regular recall. Removable restorations should be kept scrupulously clean and should be removed from the mouth for a minimum of 8 hours each day.

References

Carranza FA. Glickman's clinical periodontology. 7th ed. Philadelphia: WB Saunders, 1990:945.

Gomes BC, Renner RP. Periodontal considerations of the removable partial overdenture. Dent Clin North Am 1990; 34:653.

Renner RP, Boucher LJ. Removable partial dentures. Chicago: Quintessence Publishing, 1987:53.

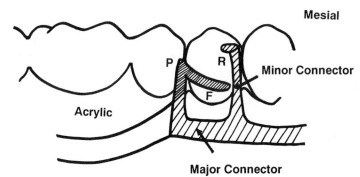

Distal

Mesial

Acrylic

Minor Connector

Major Connector

Figure 1. Illustration of a stress-releasing clasp (RPF). *R*, mesial rest; *P*, distal guide plane; *F*, circumferential clasp placed at or gingival to the tooth height of contour. The minor connector provides bracing action and is designed to cover the soft tissue minimally. The major connector is placed apical to the free gingival margin.

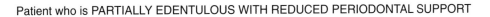

Patient who is PARTIALLY EDENTULOUS WITH REDUCED PERIODONTAL SUPPORT

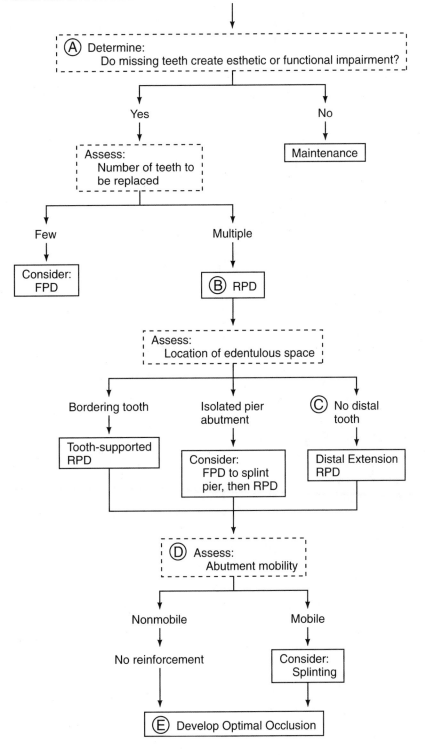

TOOTH-SUPPORTED OVERDENTURES

Robert Sarka

When diagnosis and treatment planning dictate a transition from partial edentulism to complete dentures, the remaining teeth should be evaluated for possible use as overdenture abutments. The advantages of using shortened teeth to support dentures include ridge reinforcement and preservation, retention of tactile sense and proprioception, a firm denture foundation, and generally improved denture service; however, a number of decisions must be made before determining that this type of treatment can benefit the patient.

A. Above all, candidate teeth for overdenture abutments should have a favorable prognosis. Complete dentures are indicated when the remaining teeth have a generally hopeless prognosis, but strategically located individual teeth may survive under the reduced mechanical demands of an overdenture. Restorability, lack of inflammatory periodontal disease, and feasibility of endodontic treatment are more critical factors than crown-to-root ratio, which is improved when the coronal structure is amputated and domed (after endodontic treatment to create the abutment) and mobility is reduced.

B. A number of prosthodontic factors should be evaluated. Typically, the need for denture support is greater in the mandible than in the maxilla because of reduced residual ridge and lack of seal. The dramatically atrophic ridge warrants heroic measures to preserve remaining teeth and bone; although the well-developed ridge does not require these efforts, it should be preserved with preventive prosthodontic procedures. The strategic value of the candidate teeth is determined by tooth position (canines being the most desirable), interocclusal space, and prosthodon-tic complications (e.g., large undercuts associated with retained teeth or the need to place implants in the future). The prosthodontic dentist must also determine whether the abutments will be active or passive, that is, whether they will be mechanically connected to the prosthesis by means of attachments or merely provide vertical support for the complete denture. Active abutments are under heavy stress and have more stringent requirements for root support than do passive abutments.

C. Finally, the success or failure of overdenture treatment is dependent on the patient's willingness to take responsibility for the treatment, cooperate with follow-up care, and maintain the necessary level of plaque control. Initially, the patient must tolerate endodontic treatment and periodontal therapy, including gingival grafting if insufficient attached tissue is present. A home care regimen of meticulous hygiene and daily fluoride treatment must be followed carefully. The patient needs to return to the dental office at regular intervals for evaluation and professional maintenance. Only patients with an obvious commitment to this type of dentistry should be selected.

References

Brewer AA, Morrow RM. Overdentures. St Louis: Mosby–Year Book, 1975:3, 24.

Castleberry DJ. Philosophies and principles of removable partial overdentures. Dent Clin North Am 1990; 34:589.

Zarb GA. Boucher's prosthodontic treatment for edentulous patients. 10th ed. St Louis: Mosby–Year Book, 1990:521.

A Patient Requiring DENTURES WHO HAS SEVERAL REMAINING TEETH

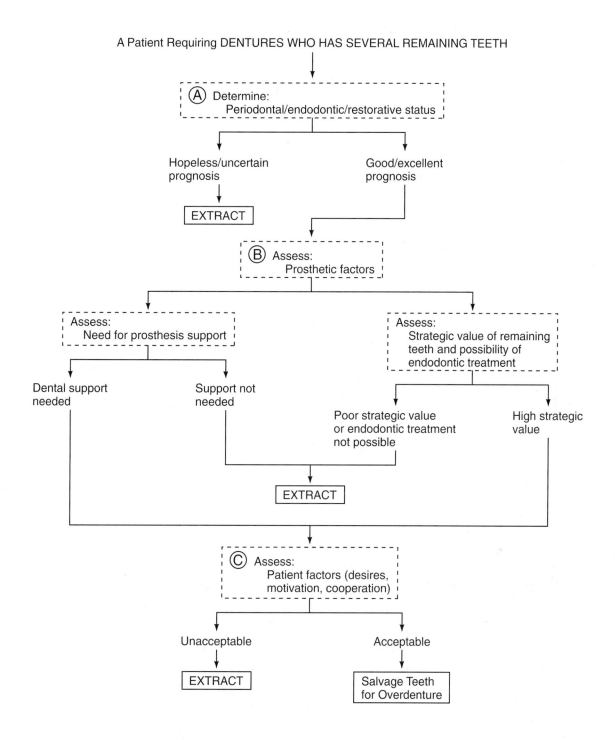

OSSEOINTEGRATED IMPLANTS FOR THE EDENTULOUS MANDIBLE OPPOSING A COMPLETE DENTURE

I. E. Naert

The rehabilitation of the edentulous mandible may be achieved by means of a fixed prosthesis or an overdenture supported by endosteal root form implants. The cumulative failure rate for prosthesis stability of Branemark implants in the mandibular symphyseal area is low (1%). Other implant systems also report good results in this area, at least for intermediate term observations. Two to six fixtures usually are placed in the interforaminal region unless the mandible is very resorbed.

A. In general, an orthopantomograph and a profile radiograph suffice for evaluation of osseous structures. When the anterior mandible height is only 7 mm and its width is limited, the use of a small number of fixtures is advised so as not to weaken the mandible and to prevent a fracture of the jawbone. In the severely resorbed mandible a very predictable procedure is the installation of two widely spaced fixtures connected above the alveolar crest by a cast bar oriented parallel to the mandibular hinge axis. The overdenture should be resilient. When loading the distal saddles of the overdenture, the fixtures should be subjected to axial loading only.

B. If there is sufficient bone volume and the patient is young, the primary choice should always be a fixed full prosthesis (for Angle Class I and II relationships). With a fixed prosthesis, bone resorption in the anterior mandible is limited to physiologic amounts. In areas distal to the fixtures, alveolar bone resorption also is minimal.

   With an Angle Class III relationship, the shortened arch destabilizes the upper denture and increases the resorption rate of the anterior maxilla. The ideal treatment is surgical correction of the Class III malocclusion by means of an osteotomy before a full fixed prosthesis is installed. A more conservative option is the placement of an overdenture, which can transfer load to the posterior area and limit overload of the anterior maxilla.

   With overdenture therapy, resorption of the posterior ridge may continue and can exceed that which occurs with a complete denture, because of the greater chewing forces associated with overdentures. Implant-supported overdentures are indicated primarily for elderly patients who do not object to a removable denture and only seek increased denture retention. To limit the harmful effects of continuous resorption of the posterior mandible, regular relining of the overdenture is indicated. This also decreases torquing forces on the fixtures.

   In the fabrication of a mandibular fixed prosthesis opposing a maxillary complete denture, the occlusal forces should be distributed over the entire maxillary arch to lower the risk of further resorption of the anterior maxilla. However, "clearing" anterior centric contacts is not recommended, because this practice may lead to overload of the distal fixtures from excessive pressure on the extension pontics.

C. It is important to distinguish between the "physiological" patient, who desires only better retention of the lower denture, and the "psychological" patient, who is not only dissatisfied with the function of the denture but also wants to be freed from "removable teeth." The clinician should carefully determine which therapy objectives are reasonable; desires for dramatically youthful appearance or social problem solving may not be realistic, and the patient may be extremely disappointed in treatment results.

References

Adell R, Eriksson B, Lekholm U. A long-term follow-up study of osseointegrated implants in the treatment of totally edentulous jaws. Int J Oral Maxillofac Implants 1990; 5:347.

Albrektsson T, Zarb G, Worthington P. The long-term efficacy of currently used dental implants. Int J Oral Maxillofac Implants 1986; 1:11.

Jemt T, Stalblad PA. The effect of chewing movements on changing mandibular complete dentures to osseointegrated overdentures: A 4-year report. J Prosthet Dent 1986; 55:357.

Naert I, Quirynen M, Theuniers G, et al. Prosthetic aspects of osseointegrated fixtures supporting overdentures: A 4-year report. J Prosthet Dent 1991; 65:671.

Quirynen M, Naert I, van Steenberghe D. Fixture design and overload influence marginal bone and fixture loss in the Branemark system. Clin Oral Impl Res, accepted for publication.

Sennerby L, Carlsson GE, Bergman B, et al. Mandibular bone resorption in patients treated with tissue-integrated prostheses and in complete-denture wearers. Acta Odontol Scand 1988; 46:135.

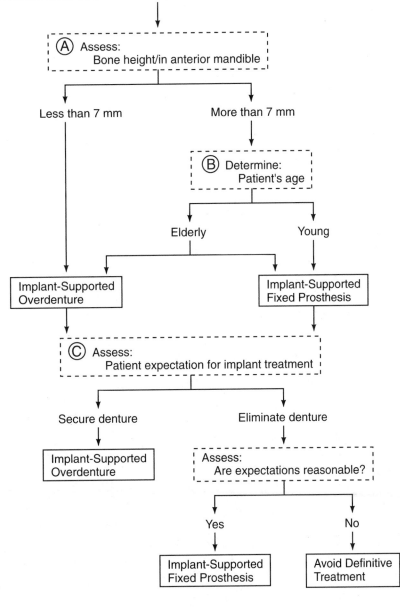

OSSEOINTEGRATED IMPLANTS FOR THE NONGRAFTED EDENTULOUS MAXILLA

I. E. Naert

A. When determining the suitability of a patient for implant treatment, physiologic factors related to looseness and discomfort of existing dentures and available bone volume must be evaluated along with psychologic factors. A patient who seeks better retention and stability for a denture may be satisfied with an implant-supported overdenture. An additional indication for a maxillary overdenture is the patient who can not tolerate coverage of the palate because of an exaggerated gag reflex. If reduction of palatal coverage eliminates retention of the conventional denture, two or four fixtures can be placed to support the denture.

The "psychological" patient is not only dissatisfied with function of the dentures but can not accept the "artificial" nature of the teeth. The clinician must distinguish patients with reasonable goals of treatment who may benefit from a full arch fixed prosthesis from those with unreasonable goals who may not be satisfied by any type of dentistry.

In the edentulous maxilla, anatomic structures such as the maxillary sinus, nasal cavity, and available bone volume influence the number of implants installed and which type of reconstruction is used. The most appropriate way to determine the amount of bone is by means of the CT scan; estimation of bone volume using an orthopantomograph is misleading, especially in the buccolingual dimension.

B. When the maxilla permits installation of at least four medium length fixtures (>10 mm), a full arch fixed prosthesis is indicated.

C. If small fixtures (7 and 10 mm) are used, a greater number of fixtures should be used to prevent overload and eventual loss; however, scientific data are still inadequate to confirm this statement.

D. In the case of Angle Class III malocclusion, whether it is congenital or developing, an osteotomy should be considered to improve jaw relationships. If the patient refuses this surgical intervention, overdentures may be required to enhance cosmetics and phonetics. For some patients an overdenture may be advantageous for prophylactic reasons also. In these situations a nonresilient overdenture supported by enough implants to carry a full arch fixed prosthesis (a fixed detachable prosthesis) should be considered.

In contrast to overdenture therapy in the lower jaw, where two unconnected fixtures seem to function well without marginal bone loss, this approach cannot be extrapolated to the maxilla. In the maxilla, when two unconnected fixtures are loaded by means of an overdenture, continuous bone loss has been detected and eventually leads to fixture loss. Long-term data are lacking to confirm a maxillary overdenture based on a limited number of fixtures (two to four) as a predictable therapy. Splinting the fixtures with a rigid cast bar may be helpful in achieving a better distribution of occlusal forces, thereby preventing overload of individual fixtures. Chewing forces should be distributed between fixtures and alveolar crest. A new configuration for resilient maxillary overdenture design is suggested.

To limit the harmful effect of continuous resorption of the posterior alveolar crest, regular relining of the overdenture should be performed to control torquing forces in the fixtures and eventual fixture loss.

References

Lothigius E, Smedberg JI, Nilnerk, et al. A new design for a hybrid prosthesis supported by osseointegrated implants: Part 1. Technical aspects. Int J Oral Maxillofac Implants 1991; 6:80.

Mericske-Stern R. Clinical evaluation of overdenture restorations supported by osseointegrated titanium implants: a retrospective study. Int J Oral Maxillofac Implants 1990; 5:375.

Patient with an UNSERVICEABLE MAXILLARY DENTURE

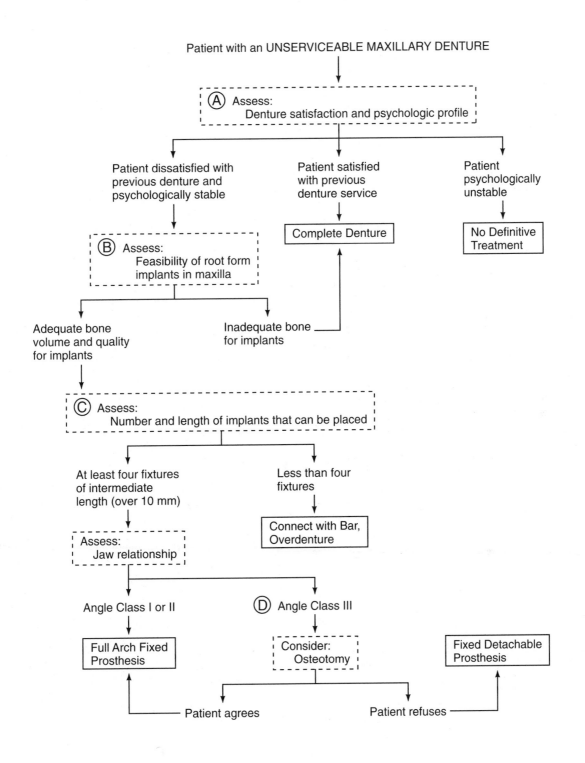

CONVENTIONAL PROSTHODONTICS VERSUS IMPLANTS FOR RESTORATION OF POSTERIOR EDENTULOUS SPACES

Jaime A. Gil-Lozano
Jaime DelRio-Highsmith
Jaime A. San Martin

In deciding whether an edentulous area would be best restored with implants or conventional fixed or removable restorations, the Kennedy classification is a useful guide. Kennedy Classes I, II, and III relate to posterior edentulous spaces.

A. For Kennedy Class I or II (bilateral or unilateral posterior distal extension cases) restorative choices are dependent on the restorative needs of the anterior abutment teeth. Whether or not they require restoration, they must have adequate existing periodontal support or be treatable periodontally. If support is good and the teeth are restorable, a combination of conventional fixed and removable prosthodontics may be employed. If the periodontal support is inadequate and adequate bone is present to support implants, teeth that will not add support to the prosthesis should be extracted and appropriate implants placed. If implants cannot be placed, a conventional denture or overdenture is indicated. If adequate implant sites are available, a fixed prosthesis based on natural teeth and/or implants may be placed. If support is inadequate for a fixed prosthesis, an implant-supported overdenture should be used.

B. If the anterior teeth do not require restoration and are periodontally sound or treatable, the adequacy of posterior bone to support implants should be assessed. Where appropriately situated implants can be placed in the posterior edentulous areas, an implant-supported fixed prosthesis can be placed. If such sites are not available or cost factors prohibit the use of implants, a conventional removable partial denture should be constructed.

C. For Kennedy Class III (posterior edentulous spaces bounded by remaining teeth) restorative choices are dependent on the restorative needs of the remaining anterior teeth. Where restorations are needed, the periodontal status should be evaluated. If the teeth are periodontally sound or treatable, a conventional full arch restoration can be placed. If the periodontal status of anterior teeth is significantly compromised, selective extraction and implant placement may be employed to create a tooth and/or implant-supported fixed prosthesis.

D. If anterior teeth are periodontally sound or treatable and do not require restoration, hopeless or useless teeth should be extracted and the adequacy of posterior abutments should be evaluated. If two or three posterior teeth are missing and only a single molar abutment remains, its periodontal status and/or treatability determines whether a conventional fixed or removable restoration is indicated. If adding implants is feasible, an implant-supported fixed prosthesis would be ideal. If inadequate bone for implants is present but the periodontal support is good, a conventional fixed prosthesis should be placed. If the periodontal support is less than adequate, a conventional removable prosthesis either clasping or just resting on the remaining molar is indicated.

E. If a second premolar and molars remain and adequate bone is present, two single implants could be placed. If the bone is inadequate to support implants but the periodontal support is adequate or treatable, a fixed prosthesis may be placed. If the periodontal status is significantly compromised, selective extraction may be employed. If an implant can be used to replace an extracted tooth, a fixed prosthesis may be placed. If support is inadequate for implant placement, a removable partial denture should be constructed.

References

Davenport JC, Basker RM, Heath JR, Ralph JP. A color atlas of removable partial dentures. London: Wolfe M.P., 1988.

Del Rio Highsmith J, Lopez Lozano JF. Fixed prostheses versus removal partial dentures. Rev Espanola de Estomatolo 1986; 34(3):191.

Eckert S, Laney W. Patient evaluation and treatment planning for osseointegrated implants. Dent Clin North Am 1989; 4:613.

Jemt T, Lekholm U, Grondahl A. A 3-year follow up study of early single implant restorations ad modum Branemark. Int J Periodont Restor Dent 1990; 10(5):341.

Martignoni M, Schonenberger A. Precision fixed prosthodontics. Chicago: Quintessence Publishing, 1990.

Parel S, Sullivan D. Esthetics and osseointegration. Dallas: Taylor Publishing, 1989.

Patient with a POSTERIOR EDENTULOUS SPACE

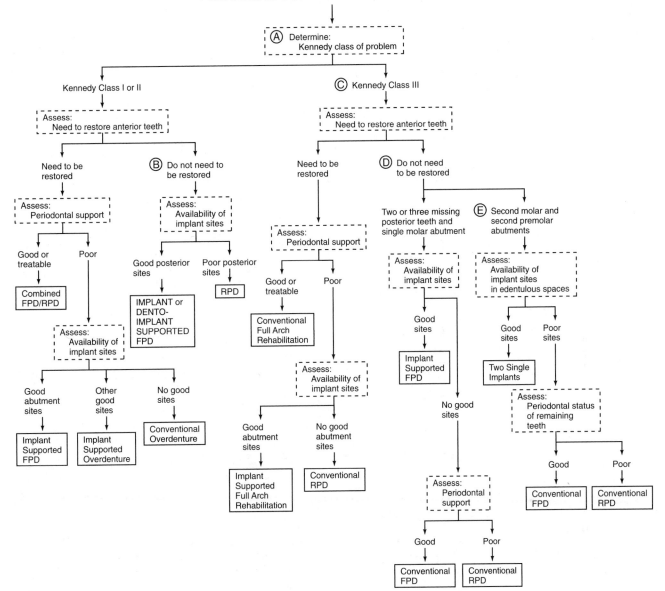

CONVENTIONAL PROSTHODONTICS VERSUS IMPLANTS FOR RESTORATION OF ANTERIOR EDENTULOUS SPACES

Jaime A. Gil-Lozano
Jaime DelRio-Highsmith
Jaime A. San Martin

A. Anterior edentulous spaces are those in Kennedy Class IV. In deciding whether to utilize implants or traditional fixed or removable prostheses to restore these spaces, the condition and number of remaining posterior teeth and the restorability and periodontal health of remaining anterior teeth must be considered.

B. Once the restorative needs of the remaining teeth have been assessed, their periodontal status must be evaluated to determine whether sufficient periodontal support remains or can be created by periodontal treatment to support the envisioned restoration. The edentulous area should be evaluated for possible implant placement. If the teeth have or can be made to have sufficient support, a fixed prosthodontic solution is preferable. Various units of natural teeth or implants may have to be included in the bridge to provide sufficient support. If sufficient support for a fixed restoration is not available, a conventional removable solution should be chosen.

C. If adequate periodontal support is not present, potential sites for implants to support a restoration should be evaluated. Hopeless or useless teeth should be identified. If implant sites are adequate and the patient so desires, an implant-supported fixed prosthesis may be constructed. If the number of teeth to be removed is excessive, an implant-supported overdenture is the treatment of choice. If the number and distribution of adequate implant sites are not favorable and the patient so desires, a conventional overdenture or denture may be the only remaining option.

D. If no need exists to restore the remaining teeth and they are periodontally healthy, treatable, or maintainable, the adequacy of potential implant sites should be assessed. If sites are adequate and their distribution permits, a fixed prosthesis based on implants and/or natural teeth can be constructed. If good sites do not exist, a removable partial denture is the treatment of choice.

References

Davenport JC, Basker RM, Heath JR, Ralph JP. A color atlas of removable partial dentures. London: Wolfe M.P., 1988.

Del Rio Highsmith J, Lopez Lozano JF. Fixed prostheses versus removal partial dentures. Rev Espanola de Estomatologia 1986; 34(3):191.

Eckert S, Laney W. Patient evaluation and treatment planning for osseointegrated implants. Dent Clin North Am 1989; 4:613.

Jemt T, Lekholm U, Grondahl A. A 3-year follow up study of early single implant restorations ad modum Branemark. Int J Periodont Restor Dent 1990; 10(5):341.

Martignoni M, Schonenberger A. Precision fixed prosthodontics. Chicago: Quintessence Publishing, 1990.

Parel S, Sullivan D. Esthetics and osseointegration. Dallas: Taylor Publishing, 1989.

Patient with an ANTERIOR EDENTULOUS SPACE

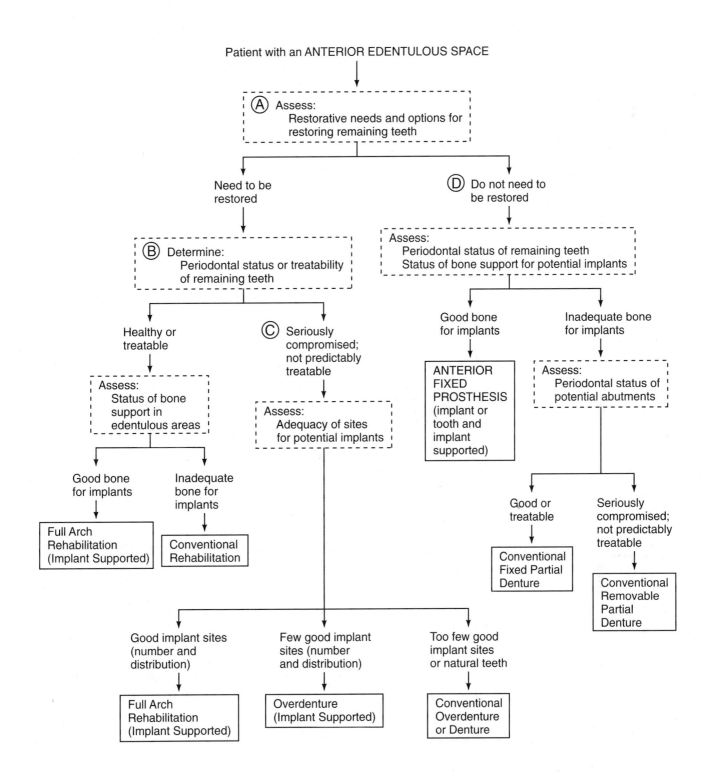

PEDIATRIC DENTISTRY

David L. Rothman, Editor

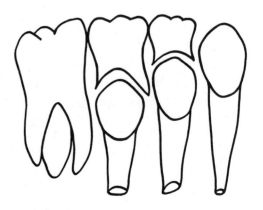

SPACE MAINTENANCE FOR FUTURE FIXED PROSTHETICS

David L. Rothman

Congenital absence of a primary or permanent tooth or the traumatic loss of a permanent tooth in a young patient requires intervention in the mixed dentition stage.

A. It must be decided if the space is to be maintained for a fixed or removable prosthesis or orthodontically closed in cases where the child may present with crowding. Multiple consultations may be necessary prior to the start of treatment. Considerations also include longevity, need for ongoing treatment, oral hygiene, and patient cooperation. Space closure may be selected if there is favorable periodontium, the mechanics of orthodontic anchorage and closure including tooth tipping and bodily movement are possible, marginal ridge heights are compatible, crowding elsewhere in the area may be alleviated by distal movement of teeth anterior to the space, and favorable factors of oral hygiene and family/caretaker support are present.

B. If space is lost and arch length is decreased, impaction or ectopic eruption of permanent teeth may occur. Two options exist, uprighting with space regaining and space closure, which both utilize active orthodontic therapy.

C. Unerupted teeth with incomplete roots in favorable angulation may erupt into extraction sites and with or without orthodontic therapy may move into a favorable, periodontally, and occlusion acceptable position. This may be attempted with early loss of first or second molars.

D. If it is determined that space maintenance for future prosthetic repair is appropriate, many factors influence selection of type of space maintainer. A thorough assessment of the young patient's periodontal status, oral hygiene, and caries indices must be made. If indications in all of the previous categories are favorable and the patient is compliant and responsible, either a fixed or removable appliance may be appropriate. If neither the young patient nor his support group appears responsible, a fixed appliance should be used. In young patients with high caries indices, removable appliances may allow the placement of topical fluoride preparations and improve the ability to perform oral hygiene techniques.

E. The decision to use a fixed or removable prosthesis depends on many of the factors discussed above. A fixed prosthesis placed in a growing patient has the potential to limit growth of the alveolus and eruption of teeth. Insertion of a fixed prosthesis is recommended in the older patient, but it may also be attempted in patients whose teeth have fully developed roots. In addition, considerations such as active participation in contact sports, esthetics, compliance, and oral hygiene all influence the decision. The use of implants in early teenaged patients is currently being investigated and may be a valid treatment option. Bonded bridges are excellent treatment options because limited preparation of abutment teeth reduces the trauma to pulps (p 218).

References

Boyd RL. New methods for chemical inhibition of plaque in orthodontic patients. In: Singer J, ed: Integrating periodontology and orthodontics. Los Angeles: University of Southern California Press, 1987:31.

Dyson JE. Prosthodontics for children. In: Wei SHY, ed. Pediatric dentistry, total patient care. Philadelphia: Lea & Febiger, 1988:259.

Evans CA, Nathanson D. Indications for orthodontic-prosthodontic collaboration in dental treatment. J Am Dent Assoc 1979; 99:825.

Hotz RP: Guidance of eruption versus serial extraction. Am J Orthod 1970; 58:1.

McDonald RE, Hennon DK, Avery DR. Managing space problems. Dentistry for the child and adolescent. 5th ed. St Louis: Mosby–Year Book, 1988:721.

Pinkham JR, Cassamassmo P, Fields H, et al: Pediatric dentistry. Philadelphia: WB Saunders, 1988:459, 495.

Child with MISSING PERMANENT TOOTH

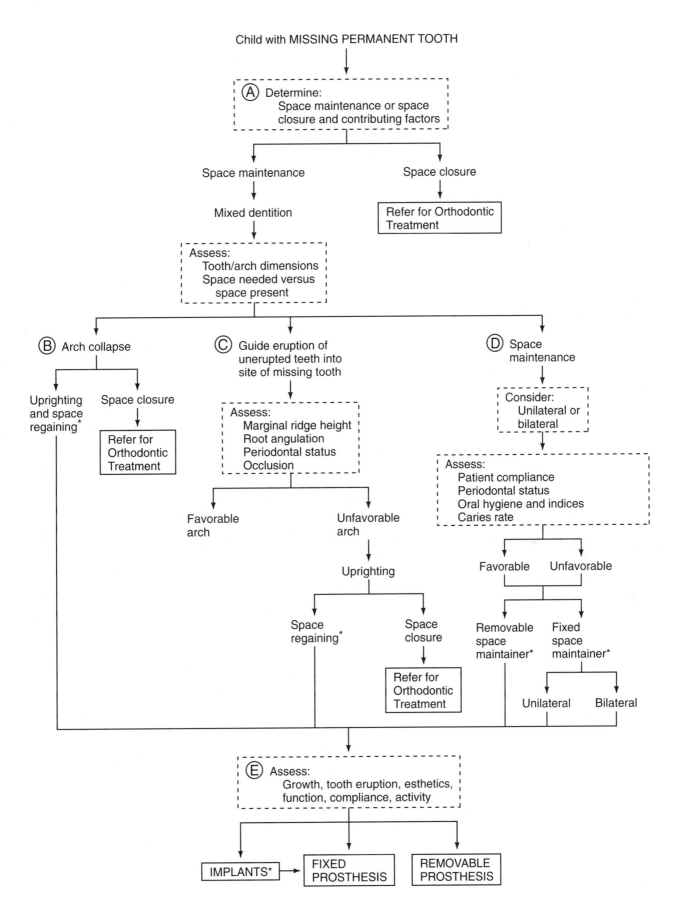

A Determine:
Space maintenance or space closure and contributing factors

Space maintenance

Space closure → Refer for Orthodontic Treatment

Mixed dentition

Assess:
Tooth/arch dimensions
Space needed versus space present

B Arch collapse

Uprighting and space regaining*

Space closure → Refer for Orthodontic Treatment

C Guide eruption of unerupted teeth into site of missing tooth

Assess:
Marginal ridge height
Root angulation
Periodontal status
Occlusion

Favorable arch

Unfavorable arch

Uprighting

Space regaining*

Space closure → Refer for Orthodontic Treatment

D Space maintenance

Consider:
Unilateral or bilateral

Assess:
Patient compliance
Periodontal status
Oral hygiene and indices
Caries rate

Favorable | Unfavorable

Removable space maintainer*

Fixed space maintainer*

Unilateral | Bilateral

E Assess:
Growth, tooth eruption, esthetics, function, compliance, activity

IMPLANTS* → FIXED PROSTHESIS | REMOVABLE PROSTHESIS

*Interim treatment.

215

TREATMENT OF IMMATURE, PULPALLY INVOLVED POSTERIOR TEETH

David L. Rothman

Immature posterior teeth may exhibit the symptoms of pulp inflammation and degeneration caused by caries. Poorly developed deep pit and fissures, poor oral hygiene, highly cariogenic diets, and low enamel resistance leads to the rapid progression of caries. Food impacted under a large operculum and inflamed gingiva may contribute because of the child's difficulty in removing debris from the area of a newly erupting tooth.

A. The treatment limiting step for pulpally involved immature teeth is the tooth's eventual restorability. If the crown of the tooth is badly damaged, the tooth may be unrestorable. If it is restorable, is there justification and compliance of the child for major endodontic and prosthetic repair? If extraction is an option, future prosthetic and space management treatment should be planned.

B. An orthodontic evaluation of the child or adolescent who needs endodontic and prosthodontic treatment is appropriate. The long-term success of the procedures is compromised by poor patient/family motivation, high caries rate, poor dental knowledge, and/or family finances.

C. Vitality testing in teeth with large pulp chamber and immature roots is not reliable. Traditionally used symptomatology of sensitivity to temperature may also be unreliable as are radiographs of incompletely formed root apices. These areas characteristically exhibit radiolucencies not representative of pulp vitality. In addition, periodontal ligaments of immature teeth appear wider on radiographs. Objective signs such as compressibility, mobility, purulence, pericoronal hyperemia with swelling, and fistulous tract formation may be the only reliable indicators. The immature tooth pulp has greater ability to heal than does the mature tooth pulp because of increased vascularity and decreased intracoronal pressure following inflammation.

D. An orthodontic evaluation in the child or adolescent who exhibits crowding is appropriate. If the patient is to be treated as an orthodontic extraction case, the option exists for removing the compromised tooth rather than the traditional premolar.

E. Apexogenesis, also known as the Frank technique, is a series of procedures that depend on vital pulp tissue to allow continued root lengthening and apical closure. Partial pulpotomy may be necessary for this procedure. Conflicting opinions exist as to whether successful completion of apexogenesis should be followed by conventional endodontic therapy.

F. Direct pulp capping implies total removal of carious material, exposing a small portion of pulp, and placing a calcium hydroxide paste over the exposure to stimulate secondary or reparative dentin. Though some believe it is important to reenter the tooth to assess whether dentin bridging has occurred, I believe this to be an unnecessary and potentially traumatizing experience for the patient and to the pulp; in my opinion permanent restoration is appropriate as is monitoring of subjective and radiographic signs.

G. Indirect pulp capping implies partial removal of carious material (leaving what is thought to be the noninfected area of dentin) and placement of a calcium hydroxide–fortified paste over the dentin. This stimulates odontoblastic formation of reparative dentin.

H. Apexification, as discussed by Cvek, is the total removal of necrotic pulp in a tooth with incompletely formed apices. Because of the wide open apex, obturation of the canals is difficult, except by surgical endodontics such as retrograde fill. In the Cvek technique calcium hydroxide is used to obturate the canals, stimulating an osteodentin bridge across the open apex. This bridge is tested at predetermined intervals (e.g., at 6 months) and the procedure continued until the bridge is complete. Conventional endodontic obturation then takes place.

References

Belanger CK. Pulp therapy for young permanent teeth. In: Pinkham JR, Fields HW, McTigue DJ, et al, eds. Pediatric dentistry: Infancy through adolescence. Philadelphia: WB Saunders, 1988:399.

Camp JH. Pedodontic-endodontic treatment. In: Cohen S, Burns RC, eds. Pathways of the pulp. 5th ed. St Louis: Mosby–Year Book, 1991:682.

Cvek M. Endodontic treatment of traumatized teeth. In: Andreason JO, ed. Traumatic injuries of the teeth. 2nd ed. Philadelphia: WB Saunders, 1981.

Frank AL. Therapy for the divergent pulpless tooth by continued apical formation. JADA 1966; 72:87–93.

Fuks AB, Bielak S, Chosale A. Clinic and radiographic assessment of direct pulp capping and pulpotomy in young permanent teeth. Pediatr Dent 1974; 4:240.

Goldman M. Root-end closure techniques, including apexifications. Dent Clin North Am 1974; 18:297.

McDonald RE, Avery DR. Dentistry for the child and adolescent. St Louis: Mosby–Year Book, 1988:435.

Young patient with an IMMATURE, PULPALLY INVOLVED POSTERIOR TOOTH

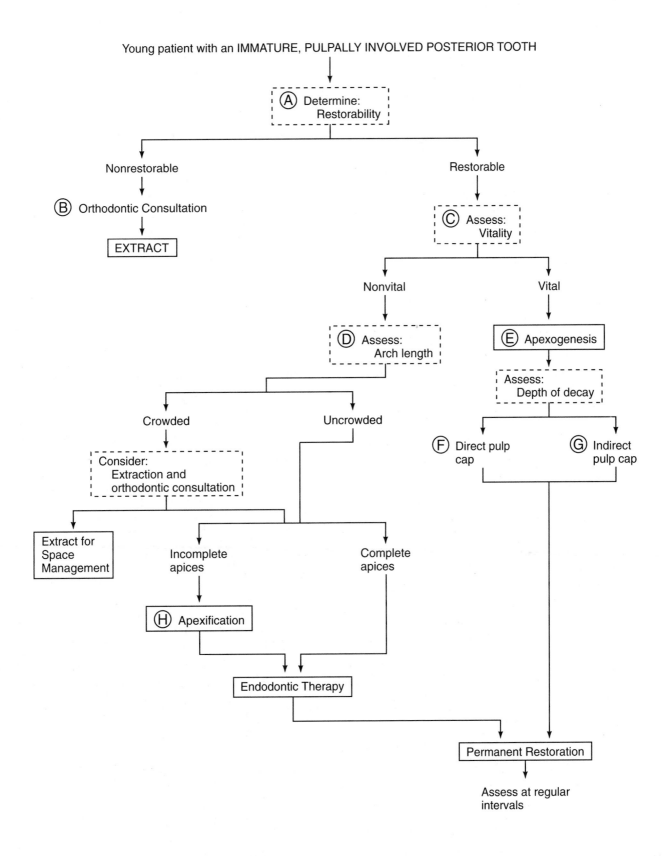

TREATMENT OF TRAUMATIZED IMMATURE ANTERIOR TEETH

David L. Rothman

Traumatic injuries to the teeth of children and adolescents are very common. In this age range males have a greater chance of injury probably because they participate in greater numbers in contact sports. An additional group of children are injured because of untreated Class II, Division I malocclusions, in which the maxillary incisors are severely proclined and unprotected by full lip coverage. Many of these injuries involve percussion, luxation, and avulsion, which damage the supporting structures. The sequelae of such injuries may include pulpal necrosis and devitalization of the tooth, dilaceration of the forming root, or total loss of the immature tooth. Nonrigid, functional splinting is a treatment option for mobile teeth with damaged periodontal structures. Teeth with root fractures require more rigid splinting for up to 6 weeks. The following discussion focuses on pulpal involvement in nondisplaced teeth that do not exhibit periodontal involvement.

A. Length of time since injury determines prognosis. In teeth with traumatically exposed pulps bacterial infection from saliva is rapid, leading to increased inflammation. Teeth with open apices appear to heal better even when exposed for longer periods because of increased vascularity. Exposure of dentin tubules following trauma also allows infection of the pulp with the usual sequelae. There are no definitive times used, rather arbitrary periods of short or long.

B. Apical closure and root length are used as markers for the pulp's ability to heal after trauma and the determination of a possibly unfavorable crown-to-root ratio in a devitalized tooth. Complete apical closure on a traumatized tooth gives a less promising prognosis. Torquing of the tooth may sever the neurovascular bundle as it enters the apical foramen. In addition, pulpal edema and extravasation of red blood cells from capillaries following injury may increase intrapulpal pressure such that the pulp autostrangulates by severing its own blood supply.

C. Type of injury, extent of damage, and loss of periodontal structures including alveolar bone and periodontal ligament must be evaluated with respect to crown-to-root ratio. If it is favorable, nonrigid splinting using light orthodontic wire, nylon fishing line, Kevlar line, or even multiple strands of floss may be appropriate.

D. Apexogenesis, or the Frank technique, is a partial pulpotomy procedure in which calcium hydroxide is placed over the pulp. This allows continued root end formation.

E. If an unfavorable crown-to-root ratio exists in a devitalized tooth, splinting may be an option but extraction is the treatment of choice with prosthetic replacement.

F. The total removal of necrotic pulp tissue in the Cvek technique of apexification allows for root end closure, not elongation, with an osteodentin type tissue. In the absence of this closure conventional endodontic therapy is difficult and surgical therapy is the only option. Calcium hydroxide paste is placed in the canal and followed radiographically. Closure is tested with a blunt probe. This procedure should not be done immediately but instead approximately 1 to 2 weeks after trauma to allow healing of the periodontal ligament and supporting structures. The calcium hydroxide can act as an irritant and has been shown to cause external resorption and ankylosis.

G. External resorption may be limited in some cases with root end closure through the use of calcium hydroxide paste placed in the canal. This is followed radiographically. The tooth may eventually be conventionally obturated.

References

Andreasen JO. Traumatic injuries of the teeth. 2nd ed. Philadelphia: WB Saunders, 1981.

Camp JH. Pedodontic-endodontic treatment. In: Cohen S, Burns RC, eds. Pathways of the pulp. 5th ed. St Louis: Mosby–Year Book, 1991:682.

Cvek M. Endodontic treatment of traumatized teeth. In: Andreason JO, ed. Traumatic injuries of the teeth. 2nd ed. Philadelphia: WB Saunders, 1981.

Frank AL. Therapy for the divergent pulpless tooth by continued apical formation. JADA 1966; 72:87–93.

Fuks AB, Bielak S, Chosale A. Clinic and radiographic assessment of direct pulp capping and pulpotomy in young permanent teeth. Pediatr Dent 1974; 4:240.

Goldman M. Root-end closure techniques, including apexifications. Dent Clin North Am 1974; 18:297.

McDonald RE, Avery DR, Lynch TR. Dentistry for the child and adolescent. St Louis: Mosby–Year Book, 1988:512.

McTigue DJ. Managing traumatic injuries in the young permanent dentition. In: Pinkham JR, Fields HW, McTigue DJ, et al, eds. Pediatric dentistry: Infancy through adolescence. Philadelphia: WB Saunders, 1988:409.

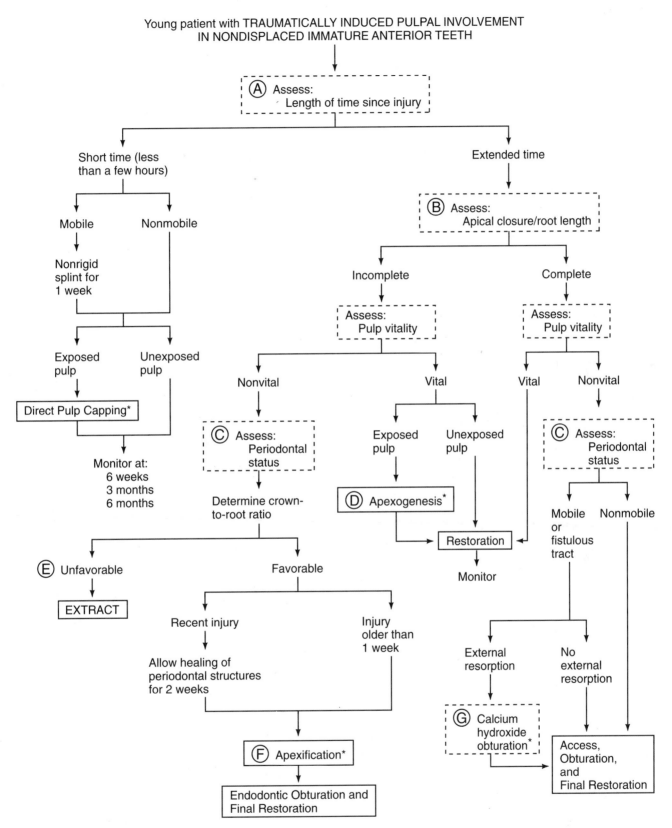

Young patient with TRAUMATICALLY INDUCED PULPAL INVOLVEMENT
IN NONDISPLACED IMMATURE ANTERIOR TEETH

(A) Assess:
Length of time since injury

Short time (less than a few hours)

Extended time

Mobile

Nonmobile

Nonrigid splint for 1 week

Exposed pulp

Unexposed pulp

Direct Pulp Capping*

Monitor at:
6 weeks
3 months
6 months

(B) Assess:
Apical closure/root length

Incomplete

Complete

Assess:
Pulp vitality

Assess:
Pulp vitality

Nonvital

Vital

Vital

Nonvital

(C) Assess:
Periodontal status

Exposed pulp

Unexposed pulp

(C) Assess:
Periodontal status

Determine crown-to-root ratio

(D) Apexogenesis*

Restoration

Mobile or fistulous tract

Nonmobile

(E) Unfavorable

Favorable

Monitor

EXTRACT

Recent injury

Injury older than 1 week

External resorption

No external resorption

Allow healing of periodontal structures for 2 weeks

(G) Calcium hydroxide obturation*

Access, Obturation, and Final Restoration

(F) Apexification*

Endodontic Obturation and Final Restoration

*Interim treatment.

219

INDEX

Page numbers in italics indicate illustrations.

Pedicle grafts, 34
  and gingival augmentation, 50
  and recession treatment, 47
  rotated, 51
Periapical radiolucency, 13, 14
Perimplantitis, 84–85
  surgical management of, 88–91
Periodontal pathogens, tests for, 20
Periodontal surgery, 92–93
  diagnosis, diagram, 93
Periodontal therapy
  and endodontic procedures, 104
  goal of, 30
  and recall visits, diagram, 95
  sequence of, 4–5
    diagnosis, diagram, 5
Periodontitis
  characteristics of, 144
  juvenile, 20
Pocket depth, diagnosis, diagram, 15, 21
Posterior teeth
  immature, pulpally involved, 216
    diagnosis, diagram, 217
  and lack of attached gingiva
    diagnosis, diagram, 161
  restorative planning for, 134–138
    diagnosis, diagram, 135
Pregnancy, 74, 106
Premolars
  extrusion, 154
  mutilated, 183
  with vertical crack, 12
Preprosthetic surgery, 196
Pritchard-type bone fill, 18, 54, 64
Pseudo-pockets, and LOA, 18
Pterygoid process, 80
Pterygomaxillary fixtures, 80
Pulmonary disease, 106
Pulpal status, 22, 194
Pulpal symptoms, diagnosis, diagram, 195, 219
Pulp chambers, 134
Pulpectomy, 102
Pulpotomy, 102

R

Radiation therapy, and implants, 72
Radicular groove
  periodontal-endodontic ramifications of, 108–111
    diagnosis, diagram, 111
Radiography, 12, 13, 66, 70, 74, 78, 84, 108, 110, 116, 138,
  156, 204
Rapid extrusion, 182–183
Recall visits
  behavioral approach to, 94–95
  and hopeless teeth, 166
  timing of, 94
Recession, 46–49, 50
  and connective tissue graft, 46
  diagnosis, diagram, 49
  and gingival augmentation, 41, 50
Referrals
  to endodontist, 106–107
  to periodontist, 6–7
    diagnosis, diagram, 7
Removable partial dentures (RPD), 180
  design considerations for, 200
  diagnosis, diagram, 197
  placement, 164
Resective surgery, 54–55, 62
Residual ridge resorption (RRR), 196
Restoration
  of anterior spaces, 210

diagnosis, diagram, 211
  endodontic effects of cast, 194
  extensive, diagnosis, diagram, 191
  following periodontal surgery, 92–93
  full coverage, diagnosis, diagram, 185
  planning, and gingival grafting, 44–45
  for posterior spaces, 208
    diagnosis, diagram, 209
  selecting individual tooth, 172
  unserviceable, diagnosis, diagram, 173, 175
Rest-proximal plate I (RPI), 38, 44
Retreatment, diagnosis, diagram, 127
Retrograde filling, 132–133
Ridge(s), 36
  augmentation, 34, 196
    deficiency, 41
  diagnosis, diagram, 37
  residual and prosthetic treatment, 196
Ridgeplasty, 36
Risk vs. benefit analysis, 98, 188
Root amputation, 62, 128–129
Root canal therapy, 114
Root end filling, 124, 132–133
Root end resection, 124, 132–133
Root extrusion, 120
Root form, 22, 24
Root perforation, 120–123
Root planing, 30, 60
Root resection, 128, 130–131
Roots, fused, 130

S

Second molars
  and impacted third molars, 16
  and partially erupted third molars, 18–19
Selective grinding
  and cracked tooth syndrome, 12, 13
  and occlusion, 178
  vs. splinting, 28–29
    diagnosis, diagram, 29
Sharpey's fibers, 160
Single-rooted teeth
  managing perforations of, 120–122
    diagnosis, diagram, 123
Sinus disease, 102
Sinus elevation, 77
Sinus grafting, 80
Sinus lift, 72
Skeletal dysplasia, 158
Space maintenance, in pediatric dentistry, 214
  diagnosis, diagram, 215
Splinting, 102
  cast restoration, 174
  determining need for, 188
  and loose teeth, 28
  and periodontal surgery, 92
  prior to surgery, 10
  and RPDs, 200
Standard of care, 104, 106
Stress-releasing clasp, 200
"Stripped perforation," 121
Subperiosteal implant, 77
Surgical endodontics, 124–125
Surgical therapy
  and crown lengthening, 32–33
  vs. maintenance, 30
    diagnosis, diagram, 31
  techniques of, 34–35
    diagnosis, diagram, 35
Supracrestal fiberotomy, 154
Supragingival margin placement, 186